In clinical tests _____
volunteers safely lost an average of 10
pounds over a period of 12 weeks. And they
did it without feeling hungry or weak. A
majority, in fact, said they were so pleased
with the diet that they would recommend it
to others.

Their extremely positive responses are
summed up by a man who lost over 60
pounds in four months: "It shouldn't be called
a diet," he says, "because you're not
depriving yourself of anything."

In a telephone survey of people who had
bought the Setpoint Diet in brochure form,
90 percent of the users said it had worked
successfully for them. They preferred it 4 to
1 over other diets they had tried. And 99
percent agreed that the Setpoint Diet is
highly nutritious and an excellent diet
overall.

SO WHAT ARE YOU WAITING FOR? YOU KNOW
THE CRASH DIETS DON'T WORK. TRY THE DIET
THAT WILL LEAVE YOU FEELING BETTER,
HEALTHIER—AND SLIMMER—FOR THE REST OF
YOUR LIFE!

# THE SETPOINT DIET
## Dr. Gilbert A. Leveille

BALLANTINE BOOKS • NEW YORK

Library of Congress Catalog Card Number: 85-90714

ISBN 0-345-32196-0

Manufactured in the United States of America

First Edition: September 1985

Cover design: Paul D. Miller

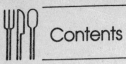

# Contents

## Note to Readers

This diet is based on the nutritional needs of the average adult. A modified version is presented for the average adolescent. The diet is not designed for use by those with special dietary needs—including children and pregnant women. If you require a special dietary regimen or have a medical history that suggests that exercise may not be advisable, consult your physician.

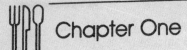

# Chapter One

# Finally—
# A Diet That Really
# Works

This is probably not the first diet book you have ever read. In fact, if you are like the one-out-of-four adult Americans who is overweight, you have probably tried many diets throughout your life. You have tried calorie-controlled diets, diets consisting of special formulas, low-carbohydrate diets, perhaps even "miracle" diets that rely on one or two foods, such as boiled eggs or grapefruit.

And, if you followed the diets as instructed, usually for two to six weeks, you probably lost weight. You were able to fit into that tight suit in time for your anniversary party, or you managed to slim down for the beach season.

Why, then, are you reading yet another diet book?

You're reading this book, I suspect, because you discovered that each of the diets you tried in the past didn't really work. Oh, they took off a few pounds, all right. But at the end of six weeks—or however long you dieted—you inevitably began to regain the weight you had lost. Sometimes you gained even more.

Or perhaps you had difficulty losing at all no matter how faithfully you followed a diet. You endured hunger pangs, weakness, and boredom yet failed to shed more than a pound or two. If so, you are not alone: It is a

1

common experience to follow a diet to the letter and yet fail to lose a meaningful amount of weight.

No matter what your experience, when any diet failed to give you lasting slimness, the chances are you felt guilty. "I'm a glutton," you told yourself. "I just don't have any willpower."

For many years it was the accepted belief that failure to lose weight was somehow a moral failing—that the unsuccessful dieter was lacking in willpower and motivation. However, research over the last thirty years has gradually proved this just isn't so. In fact, we now have evidence to the contrary: The truth is that willpower alone will not enable you to lose weight and keep it off.

Or, to put it another way: It is almost impossible to take weight off for good simply by eating less.

I learned all this myself from hard experience. From the time I was a teenager I had a problem controlling my weight. Just like you, I tried all the diets. And like you, I always lost a few pounds at first and then gained them all back.

I had the misfortune to be overweight at a time when medical and scientific opinion said that people were over-weight because they were gluttons. Even though I didn't seem to eat more food than my slimmer friends, I felt guilty.

Then I started looking at the problem in a different light. If I couldn't control my gluttony, I reasoned, I would have to try to burn more calories. And so, when I was a senior in high school, I started running.

Almost immediately I began to lose weight. Over the next five to ten years, I always regained pounds when for some reason I stopped exercising, and my weight wouldn't come down until I began to exercise again.

Was exercise the key? And if so, how did the key fit? Through reading I discovered that scientific opinion did not completely explain my observations. Running two miles, for example, burns 200 calories. Since I ran two miles every day, that was a deficit of 1400 calories per week, which should have amounted to approximately ½-pound weight loss per week. But even without dieting, I lost weight more rapidly when I first began my program. And gradually, without change in my eating or running habits, my weight had stabilized at a new lower level. According to the accepted reasoning of the day—based on a limited understanding of exercise's effect—I should not have lost weight as quickly as I did. And I should not have stabilized at the new, lower weight when I was apparently still burning an extra 1400 calories per week; I should have continued to lose weight.

I could not deny my own observations. But neither could I ignore that my experience seemed to be contradicting what scientists were saying at that time. It was partly because of my interest in this seeming paradox that I entered the field of nutrition research.

Only in recent years have scientists finally begun to fit the pieces of the puzzle together. It is now known that the traditional arithmetical model of dieting—that the number of calories taken in must be balanced by an equal number of calories of energy expenditure—is only part of the story when it comes to weight loss. Though correct as far as it goes, this model doesn't take into account individual differences in the rate at which calories are burned just to maintain living processes, such as breathing and digestion. The truth is that we devote 50 percent or more of our energy output to those processes alone. It was long believed that the rate at which we burn energy for these purposes was constant and couldn't be changed—but now we know that isn't so. This new information forms the foundation of what we now call "setpoint theory."

Simply put, your setpoint is the weight that your body will try to maintain no matter how many calories—within limits—you take in. In other words, your body actively resists any attempts to lose (or gain) weight. No wonder traditional diets don't work in the long run! They missed the key point: *The only way you can lose weight and keep it off is to lower your setpoint.* Just lowering your caloric intake isn't enough.

Working with a team of dietitians and physiologists and relying on the latest medical research, I have created a dieting plan that can lower your setpoint—and solve, once and for all, your chronic weight problem.

The Setpoint plan is not an ordinary "calorie-restricted" diet. It is, in fact, far more than just a weight-loss plan. Setpoint is a positive way of eating and living that will leave you feeling better—and, by the way, healthier. If you want to lose weight, you will—and then you will be able to keep the weight off while maintaining a balanced, nutritious diet and an active life. In addition, by following Setpoint principles, you can also improve the healthfulness of the way you (and your family) now eat and live— even if you are *not* interested in losing weight.

Unlike ordinary diets, the Setpoint plan allows you to eat moderate amounts of literally anything you want, including many foods—such as desserts and alcoholic beverages—that are forbidden on most calorie-restricted diets. And yet, unlike all those restrictive diets—many of which do not give you balanced nutrition—the Setpoint Diet provides all the vitamins, minerals, protein, and other nutrients that you need for optimal health. Setpoint allows you to lose weight steadily at a safe and healthy rate: 1 to 3 pounds a week. It also provides enough flexibility to fit comfortably into any life-style for a lifetime.

In clinical tests of the Setpoint Diet, volunteers safely lost an average of 18 pounds over a period of 12 weeks. And they did it without feeling hungry or weak. A majority, in fact, said they were so pleased with the diet that they would recommend it to others. Their extremely positive responses are summed up by a man who lost over 60 pounds in 4 months: "It shouldn't be called a diet," he says, "because you're not depriving yourself of anything."

We at General Foods offered the basic Setpoint Diet to the American public in brochure form in April 1984, and within a year more than 250,000 people had purchased copies. A telephone survey by National Family Opinion, Inc., measured purchaser reaction to the diet in the fall. More than 400 purchasers around the nation were contacted. Of those who had already used the diet, 90 percent said it had worked successfully for them! They preferred it 4-to-1 over other diets they had tried. And 99 percent agreed that the Setpoint Diet is highly nutritious and an excellent diet overall.

The Setpoint plan is not a "miracle" diet. It will not give you instant, eternal thinness with no effort. It does require some commitment and some planning on your part, including some simple changes in your daily life.

But it may *seem* like a miracle, because if you follow this plan, you will lose weight gradually and safely, you should never be hungry, you will feel more energetic than you ever did before. Best of all, you will be able to keep that weight off for a lifetime.

In the next chapter we'll see how setpoint theory works and what it can do for you.

# Chapter Two

# Setpoint Theory: The Reality of Dieting

## Why Other Diets Don't Work

Everything I told you in the preceding chapter may seem too good to be true. After all, if other diets don't work, why should the Setpoint Diet be any different?

There's an old saying in the medical community: If there are numerous "cures" for any given problem, it means that none of them works! There are many, many diet "cures" on the market, and—it's true—they seldom work long-term. As you will see, however, Setpoint is different. Before explaining why the Setpoint Diet can succeed, let us take a look at the reasons why other diets do not work in the long run—and why they may even be dangerous.

First, you probably know that your body relies on three basic substances for energy and repair: fats, proteins, and carbohydrates. Fat, which includes oils, butter, and animal fat, is a very concentrated form of energy. It is stored in the muscles, around certain organs, and just under the skin (where any excess can become visible as flab!). Our bodies have learned through evolution to become expert at storing fat as a defense mechanism. When food isn't readily available, the fat can be withdrawn from fat cells and burned for energy.

Carbohydrates, which include sugars, grains, and starchy foods, are used to meet the immediate energy requirements of your body, including your brain. Your body cannot store carbohydrates as such, except in very small amounts (mostly in the muscles and liver). An excess of carbohydrate beyond your current energy needs is turned into fat and stored in that form.

Proteins, whose richest sources include meats, dairy products, and legumes, are the basic building blocks of your body. Their constituent parts, amino acids, are used to build and repair body cells. Under normal circumstances, any excess amino acids not used for building body protein are available for energy if needed and, like carbohydrates, lead to additional fat if not needed.

Your body depends on all three of these substances to run efficiently, and going on any diet that eliminates or severely cuts back on any one of them is asking for trouble. Unfortunately, many popular diets overemphasize only one or two of them. This can not only be dangerous; it is ultimately self-defeating and inevitably makes any weight problem worse. To see why, let's take a closer look at some of the most popular types of diets.

One classic form of the fad diet emphasizes only one or two nutrients or groups of nutrients (such as proteins or fats). These are doomed to failure since they do not change your long-term habits—habits that helped make you overweight in the first place. Typical of this sort of plan is the low-carbohydrate diet, which, in many guises, has been around for years.

The low-carbohydrate diet has long been popular because it seems to produce very rapid weight loss. Since it emphasizes only fats and proteins, your ready stores of carbohydrate are quickly depleted, and with them goes the water that held them in the cells. Naturally this tends to produce a quick weight loss, but most of that loss is water, not fat. And once the water is gone, your rate of weight loss slows down also.

Fine, you say; but once the carbohydrate stores are gone, won't the body begin to use fat for energy? The answer is yes, but unfortunately it is not so simple as that. On any very low carbohydrate diet, once you have used up your stored carbohydrates, your body does begin to use fat for energy. But fat cannot be converted to glucose (sugar), which is needed at all times by certain body tissues, including your brain. Thus, once your stores of carbohydrate are gone, your body has to look elsewhere for the sugar it needs. It has no choice but to withdraw protein from your muscle cells and use that protein to make its own sugar. In a way, your body is literally "eating itself," destroying muscle tissues, which may be one cause of the weakness many people experience on this sort of diet.

Furthermore, because oxidation ("burning") of protein creates waste by-products, water from your body tissues will be called upon by the kidneys to help flush the wastes from the body. Again, this will seem to produce more weight loss, but again, it is in the form of water, not fat. As soon as you go off the diet and begin eating carbohydrates again, as you eventually will *have* to do, you will replace that water as quickly as you lost it. Such a diet will result in the loss of some fat but will also result in a loss of lean muscle tissue; even more discouraging, it will cause you to regain rapidly the weight you have lost.

A final note of warning: Not only are low-carbohydrate diets ineffective—they can be dangerous to your health. They are deficient in a number of nutrients, most notably the B vitamins. There is also evidence that they may be stressful to the heart and kidneys.

Other diets, such as a recent one that emphasized eating large quantities of fruit, also work primarily by promoting diuresis (loss of water). These diets, too, are ineffective and potentially dangerous. Not only is your body not receiving all the nutrients it needs, but also the chemical balance of sodium and potassium can be disturbed, affecting the action of all your muscles, including your heart. Such a diet may not do any harm for a short while, but it does not change long-term eating behavior and will not keep weight off for any significant period of time.

Another popular diet is the fast, or the modified fast, which seem to produce dramatic results in a very short period of time, in much the same way as a low-carbohydrate diet. Ed H., a 46-year-old chemist, goes on such a diet periodically whenever he feels he wants to lose 10 pounds or so. "It's great," he says. "Once I lost nine pounds in four days taking in nothing but coffee and vitamins." What Ed does not acknowledge is that this "diet" is not only dangerous, depriving the body of needed nutrients, but it's also totally ineffective: if it truly worked, he would not need to go on it so often. Furthermore, by the end of the fasting period, he admits to feeling weak and out of sorts, and he inevitably regains most of the weight within a day or two—not surprising, since it was nearly all water that he lost!

The truth is that *no diet*, including the Setpoint Diet, can promise you a weight loss of more than 5 pounds of *fat* per week.

I cannot emphasize this too strongly. No matter how overweight you are, there is a limit to how much fat weight (as opposed to water weight) you can lose. Even if you went on a complete fast, the maximum amount of fat you could lose in a week is 5 to 7 pounds—and in the vast majority of cases it would be much less. All the rest would be water loss, and all of it would return as soon as you went off the diet.

Finally, there are many balanced, calorie-controlled diets on the market, offered both in books and by diet groups. These diets emphasize a balance of nutrients, and as far as they go, they are fine. But even these, and particularly the very low calorie plans (below 1200 calories a day), are doomed to failure, because they are based on the misunderstood arithmetical model of dieting and weight control mentioned in chapter 1.

Don't get me wrong. These diets have been created by well-meaning experts relying on the best information that was available to them at the time. The history of science is full of stories of hypotheses that seemed to explain things for a time but were later proven wrong as new, better theories took their place. While the old "calorie balance" theory is a central part of the story, it is still only *part* of the story. The rest has to do with individual differences—and with the ability of the body itself to maintain its weight within set limits.

## What Happens When You Diet

I mentioned earlier that fat is an efficient way of storing energy for the long haul and that your body does everything it can to hold on to those stores of fat. This is only one of a number of mechanisms through which the body tends to *defend its weight*. This means that through different physiological and psychological mechanisms the body actively resists any gain or loss of weight.

You have probably noticed this yourself: No matter how overweight you are, whether a little or a lot, it often takes a great deal of overeating—or of dieting—to make a noticeable difference in what you weigh. (I'm not talking about a temporary gain of, say, 2 pounds the day after an exceptionally big meal.) This tendency of the body to defend its weight applies to all humans, regardless of whether they are overweight or underweight.

Most of these weight-defense mechanisms are thought to have developed in ancient times, when the supply of food was uncertain. And they are potent—they were developed, after all, to insure survival. Thus, in times of famine, those who were very good at holding onto their stores of fat would survive and pass the trait on. In pre-historic times this was useful; today it is a liability. According to some studies, an adult who has been obese (people are considered obese if extra fat causes them to be 25 percent or more above the weight listed for their height in the chart on p. 34) since childhood can cut calories to fewer than 1000 per day and, apart from water loss, still not lose weight for up to 6 weeks! Likewise, in experiments, naturally lean adults have doubled their food intake for as much as 6 weeks without significant weight gain.

How does the body manage to hold on to its weight so tenaciously? One of the most important psychological mechanisms is intense hunger. As soon as your body senses that you are not taking in enough calories to remain at your present weight, it sends out hunger pangs telling you so. This is the reason so many people find that they are always hungry when on a diet.

The physiological mechanisms by which the body maintains itself are more numerous and more complex. One ability that the body developed early on was that of automatically slowing down or speeding up the rate at which it used calories for energy, depending on how much food was available.

Your basal metabolic rate is the rate at which you burn calories just to stay alive—your "resting rate." Whenever you perform an activity, the total amount of energy you expend is equal to your resting rate *plus* the number of calories required by the activity. Thus, people with a lower rate use less energy in the performance of a task (or in doing nothing at all) than people with a higher rate. Your skinny neighbor may actually be burning more calories all day long—whether he is napping or mowing the lawn—than you are when you do the exact same things for the exact same amounts of time.

Research now shows that when you cut down on calories *your basal metabolic rate actually declines*; that is, the amount of energy that you use just for living is reduced. This means that when you start dieting, you actually start burning fewer calories than you would have before. Thus, for many dieters, the very act of dieting can make it increasingly difficult to lose weight.

The tendency of the body to maintain its weight also helps to explain the well-known "plateau effect" in which a dieter may reach a new weight level and then get stuck there. Your body has simply adjusted to a lower basal metabolic rate in order to maintain itself. For example, if you go on a diet that reduces your calorie intake by 500, your body soon learns to maintain itself on 500 fewer calories than usual—the natural response to starvation. Studies show that this adjustment can begin as early as *24 to 48 hours* after the reduced calorie intake begins!

This theory also helps to explain why so many people tend to regain lost weight very quickly: now that your body has learned to get along on, say, 1000 calories a day, if you go off a diet and start eating more, you start putting on fat. Your body eventually will increase its metabolic rate so you'll stop gaining—but too late! You'll be right back where you started!

For many "yo-yo" dieters, there is evidence that the basal metabolic rate never returns completely to its pre-diet level, so you can end up weighing even more than before. Worse than that, some studies indicate that repeated dieting can actually train your body to reduce its basal metabolic rate more and more rapidly each time—and then to regain lost weight just as quickly.

Thus it seems clear that dieting by calorie reduction alone is doomed to fail—and it is. *But the good news is that there is a remarkable and simple solution to long-term weight control.*

## Dieting and Your Setpoint

We have seen that through various mechanisms the body actively works to keep its weight at a near-constant level, whether that is fashionably slim or uncomfortably overweight. This weight that the body generally tries to maintain is known as the weight setpoint.

Actually our weight setpoint is only one of many physiological setpoints—body temperature is another, as is the balance of certain chemicals in our body fluids. A setpoint is simply a narrow range within which your body works to maintain the most efficient balance. Without ever thinking about it, your body will signal you to do what you must to remain in balance, or homeostasis.

Thus, with your temperature setpoint, your body automatically adjusts to increased environmental temperature by producing sweat so evaporation can cool you off. When it is cold, you may respond by shivering, which produces muscular heat. Not everyone has exactly the same setpoint for any bodily function, but most setpoints, for most people, are very similar. For example, people do vary in their body temperature from the standard of 98.6 degrees, but not by very much.

Weight setpoint, on the other hand, does vary widely from person to person. Some people who are blessed with very low setpoints can eat virtually anything they want and not gain weight, because the excess is burned off immediately. Others, cursed with a higher setpoint, find that it is nearly impossible to lose weight, because the body will actively conserve all the energy coming in to keep the body at that weight.

Why haven't you been told this before? Well, for years most doctors and scientists didn't realize that dieting itself affects the basal metabolic rate. It took a great deal of research to prove that the energy equation was more complicated than simply walking one mile to make up for eating a 100-calorie apple.

Second, the idea of a setpoint for weight was initially rejected because there is such a wide variation in human weights, unlike the relatively constant human temperature. If there were a weight setpoint, scientists reasoned, it must be a very ineffective or feeble one. Otherwise why would the normal weight of one human vary from that of another by as much as hundreds of pounds? Also, because of this wide variation, it was impossible to measure setpoint the way you can measure temperature. Nonetheless, countless experiments with rats and humans have demonstrated that there is indeed a weight setpoint for each individual, although this is not fixed throughout life or under all circumstances.

You can get a rough idea of your own present setpoint by asking yourself how much you generally weigh when you are not consciously paying attention to how much you eat: This is your setpoint. Whenever you try to deviate from this setpoint, as with calorie-reduced dieting, biological forces come into play and work to hold your weight at its setpoint level. This is also true even if you try to gain weight—experiments have shown that it is very difficult to make naturally lean people obese.

# What Setpoint Means to You

In practical terms, setpoint theory explains a great many things that may have been troubling you for a long time.

For one thing, it explains why dieting is so difficult and ultimately ineffective—your body has been sabotaging your every effort to lose weight. When you cut calories, your body adjusts through reduced expenditure, stranding you on plateaus where you lose little or no weight.

Second, it explains why you can't keep weight off *after* a diet. Your body, convinced that it has been living in lean times, quickly tries to put back on as much weight as it has lost.

Third, setpoint theory explains why we tend to gain weight with age even though we have not increased our intake of food. The setpoint is not necessarily static— that is, it can change in response to a number of things (and we will see more about this in the next chapter). One thing that can change your setpoint is aging. It is known, for example, that from about the age of twenty onward, our basal metabolic rate slows by as much as 10 percent per decade. If you continue at the same activity level, even without eating more, you will start to gain weight.

Fourth, setpoint theory explains why so many people, even those who are obviously overweight, are hungry all the time and have only to "look at a cookie" to gain weight. Current research indicates that many such dieters, because of social pressure or warnings from their doctors, constantly monitor their weight and keep it at a level that is probably lower than their actual setpoint. Thus, they are in a chronic state of semistarvation, as far as their bodies are concerned, even though they may actually be many pounds overweight. A study has shown that many obese people exhibit some of the same psychological and physiological traits as victims of actual starvation: constant hunger, a tendency to eat very quickly, and a marked craving for sweets and other palatable foods.

All of this—our efficiency at storing fat, the tendency

of the body to lower basal metabolic rate in response to calorie reduction, the intense hunger pangs by which the body tries to tell you it is starving—explains why ordinary diets simply cannot work in the long term. It is obvious that they are doomed to ineffectiveness unless the setpoint can somehow be changed.

## The Good News: How the Setpoint Diet Can Help

The Setpoint Diet helps you change your setpoint. It is actually a combination plan that will help you lose weight while you lower your setpoint, thus helping you keep the weight off. It consists of two parts, which should be followed together: a moderate reduction in calories that allows you to eat a variety of foods in balance and moderation, and an exercise plan, which also emphasizes balance, variety, and moderation.

This combination is important because the only known safe way to lower your setpoint is to perform moderate exercise daily. This is not as onerous as it sounds: in fact, it can be enjoyable. In the next chapter we will take a look at how exercise works to lower your setpoint and what we mean by moderate exercise.

# Chapter Three

# The Diet-Exercise Connection

More than one expert in the field of obesity treatment has speculated that our highly mechanized modern way of life may be the primary cause of obesity—as Tufts University president Jean Mayer puts it, "an inactive life for man is as recent and as abnormal as cages are for animals." In primitive times, any caveman who was inactive a great deal of the time did not live long; most of our ancestors were constantly on the move, foraging or hunting for food, running from predators, moving from one area to another just to survive. Our hunger-control mechanisms developed in response to this way of life, and some research indicates that inactivity may, in fact, interfere with these controls. Inactivity itself seems in many cases to be a kind of appetite stimulant, indicating a breakdown in the body's quest for energy balance.

So strong is the connection between inactivity and obesity that many experts now feel that in general "overweight equals underexercise." Studies show, for example, that overweight individuals of all ages move less for any given activity than their leaner counterparts throughout the day—heavy people were even found in one study to spend an extra hour a day in bed! It becomes a vicious cycle: inactivity leads to obesity, which leads to further inactivity, increasing the obesity. Yet an increase in activity itself can create a dramatic change.

Louise L., a writer, is a good example of how adding activity can make a change. She had been sedentary her whole life ("Even as a kid I was a slug"); by the age of 30, her weight had crept up to near 140—20 pounds more than she had weighed in college. Finally—when she developed high blood pressure—her doctor put her on an exercise program consisting of walking and slow jogging. Within a few months her blood pressure was down, but even more important, "So was my weight. I didn't really eat any less. It just happened. And even better, the weight stayed off, even when I would go to a party and binge on food. It was like a miracle."

Like Louise, many dieters have discovered this "miracle," which isn't really a miracle at all. Instead, it simply means that regular, moderate exercise over a period of weeks had lowered Louise's weight setpoint. Over the years, her weight setpoint had increased from 120 to 140. Exercise brought it down again to 120; that's now the weight that her body tries to maintain and, barring any unusual changes in her diet or life-style, it will stay at that level—as long as she continues her moderate exercise.

## How Exercise Lowers the Setpoint

Experts don't agree on exactly how exercise works to lower the setpoint, but all studies show that it does. What we do know is that regular exercise helps you to lose weight by somehow enlisting your body to work with you and not against you.

As we have seen, your body strives to maintain your setpoint through a number of potent physiological mechanisms. Moderate daily exercise acts to counter these mechanisms in at least five ways:

◊ First, it burns calories;

◊ Second, it actually speeds up the rate at which you burn calories around the clock—that is, it speeds up your basal metabolic rate;

◊ Third, it burns fat and builds lean tissue;

◊ Fourth, it helps you to "waste calories" after a meal, burning up the excess that you don't need; and

◊ Fifth, it reduces your appetite.

Let's take a look at each of these mechanisms in turn.

It is obvious that exercise does burn calories; jog two miles and use up 200 calories. You may see this figure and become discouraged, thinking, "If I have a candy bar, I will have to run two miles to work it off." But if you were to walk or jog two miles every single day, you would use an extra 1400 calories every week—which in two weeks can add up to almost a pound of fat! Furthermore, you needn't jog that two miles. You can walk or run it at any speed, and it will still add up to around 100 calories per mile—a pretty fair exchange for a small amount of work. But burning calories is only part of the reason that exercise helps you lose weight and keep it off. Don't forget that exercise works in other ways, too.

The most exciting news for all dieters is that recent research indicates that your basal metabolic rate (BMR) is actually elevated for up to forty-eight hours after exercise. Remember that the BMR is the rate at which you use energy just for living; it accounts for 50 percent or more of all the energy you expend during the day. Thus, if you exercise regularly and so raise your basal metabolic rate, calories will be burned at a faster rate while you are doing your other everyday activities—or even sleeping! Your exercise is actually giving you a double benefit— not only is it burning calories while you perform it, but it is kicking you into high gear at all other times.

Third, exercise helps to build lean tissue (muscle), which results in a slimmer, healthier look as fat is lost and muscle mass is increased. Lean tissue itself has a higher metabolic rate than fat tissue—meaning it takes more calories to maintain. The more muscle you have, then, the more tissue you have that burns calories at an elevated rate. A further note: Since muscle weighs more than fat but takes up less space, a dieter can actually lose inches without losing weight. It is a common experience for exercisers initially to report that they have dropped one or two clothing sizes without an appreciable weight loss showing up on the scale.

Recent studies show that physically fit individuals are better able to handle large meals than unfit people. That is to say that if a fit woman eats a particularly large meal, her body will "waste" the extra calories, whereas a less fit person will store more of those calories as fat. This effect is known as *dietary-induced thermogenesis*, and some studies show that fit people are able to "waste" twice as many calories as sedentary people.

Finally, moderate exercise actually lowers your appetite. Many dieters are afraid to exercise because they believe that exercise will increase their appetite. In fact, the exact opposite is the case: Current research, as well as the experience of countless exercisers, indicates that an ongoing program of *moderate* exercise seems to reduce hunger, even on those days when the subject doesn't exercise.

This may seem to fly in the face of your own experience. If you are generally sedentary—getting most of your exercise by, say, walking to the bus stop—you may have noticed that an occasional game of tennis or even a period of working in the garden can leave you ravenous. It is also true that extremely heavy exercise, such as a day of hiking, can increase your appetite temporarily. The difference, however, is that neither occasional moderate exercise—such as that tennis game—nor heavy exercise has the appetite-reducing effect I am talking about. For that, only daily, moderate exercise works. Each element must be present for the exercise to lower your appetite: It must be performed *regularly* (daily or nearly so), and it must be *moderate* (neither too light nor too strenuous).

The conclusions of studies on exercise and appetite are indicated in the graph on page 20, which shows the relationship between appetite (measured by calorie intake per day) and various levels of physical activity.

All of the physiological effects described above combine to help lower your setpoint and make the Setpoint Diet really work. As a kind of bonus, however, there is a sixth, psychological way in which carrying out a regular program of exercise can guarantee success: It reduces tension and improves self-esteem as you begin to see what you have accomplished. This is particularly true if you have been inactive for a number of years. Not only can this psychological lift help to reduce some of the nervous causes of overeating, but it also may provide an incentive to continue the program.

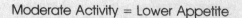

Moderate Activity = Lower Appetite

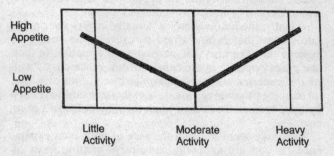

Representative chart shows relationship between appetite (measured by calorie intake per day) and various levels of physical activity.

How much exercise is needed to help you turn up your body's fires and melt away excess pounds? Less than you might think! Current research indicates that a program of light and moderate activities performed continuously for only a half hour a day is enough to permanently lower your setpoint and help you lose weight and keep it off.

## What Is Moderate Exercise?

If you are like many "confirmed nonexercisers," you may quail at the thought of exercising a half hour a day. It sounds like a lot of time and effort. Perhaps you've even tried to exercise before but couldn't stick with it.

I can sympathize with your misgivings. But if you are truly serious about losing weight once and for all, and keeping it off, than I urge you to read on. I can't promise that you will find an exercise program effortless. But I can assure you that if you give it a fair chance you will not only lose weight; you will begin to feel better than you have in years. You will probably even come to find, as have many Setpointers, that the half hour you spend in physical activity can be an enjoyable part of your daily life.

First, let's take the time commitment. One half hour a day adds up to only three-and-a-half hours a week—probably less time than you spend watching television or reading the papers. Furthermore, a good part of that exercise time can be used to do something you would be doing anyway—such as walking (although under Setpoint you may have to do it faster). And besides, you will soon discover that the exercise time will make you feel so good that you won't want to do without it.

What do I mean by moderate exercise? First of all, it is activity that makes your heart beat faster—but not too fast—and in which you may begin to perspire. Second, it is one that you can perform continuously. A good example of a moderate exercise is walking. I'm not talking about the sort of walking you already do in daily life. To lower your setpoint, you must walk briskly, fast enough to raise your heart rate and get you breathing faster, and you must do it for thirty minutes continuously. If, on the other hand, you dawdle along the street, stopping to look in store windows, it's not strenuous enough—you will burn some calories, but you will not condition your body and begin to lower your setpoint.

Now, think about your daily activities. What activity do you already do that could be incorporated into the Setpoint plan?

If done continuously and vigorously enough, all of the following could be part of your exercise plan: mowing the lawn, waxing the floors, jumping rope, climbing stairs, raking leaves. Recreational activities might include aerobic dancing, ice skating, squash, rowing, basketball. The key is to perform the activities at a high enough level so your heart rate rises and your breathing speeds up, and to perform them continuously for thirty minutes. (More specific information on exercising appears in chapter 6.)

It is the idea of performing the exercise continuously that seems to lead to some confusion. I am often told by women with small children at home, "I don't need any more exercise—I'm chasing two kids all day," or, "After picking up after my three-year-old I'm too tired to do anything else." I can sympathize with these women— taking care of small children *is* exhausting. And certainly all that walking and bending over does burn calories. But it's mostly stop-and-go, intermittent exercise. It doesn't really train the body to the point where the setpoint is lowered. All current research indicates that in order for the setpoint to be affected the activity must last for 30 consecutive minutes.

Don't let this news discourage you. You don't have to do the same exercise every day—or even the same exercise for the entire 30 minutes. For example, one day you could dance to a favorite record for 15 minutes and then walk briskly around the neighborhood afterward. The next day go bike riding before dinner. You needn't ever do an exercise that you don't like. The key is to work out regularly and continuously.

## Why Exercise and Diet Must Be Combined

"All right," you say, "maybe I will try exercising for a while, just to see what happens. But if exercise does all these wonderful things, why do I still have to diet?"

Well, the truth is that you may *not* have to diet. If you have a very small amount of weight to lose—say five pounds—regular, moderate exercise alone should do the job for you. But for many dieters, especially those who have more than a very few pounds to lose, exercise alone is simply too slow.

Studies have shown that the quickest, safest, and most effective way to lose fat while maintaining lean tissue is to combine exercise with calorie reduction. The two go hand in hand to make your body work with you: While dieting alone lowers your basal metabolic rate, exercise raises it, so that the fewer calories you are eating on the diet are burned at a higher rate than they would be if you were only dieting. Also, since exercise helps to reduce your appetite, this counters your body's "starving" response produced by lower calorie intake.

# Other Benefits of Exercise

Juanita Rivas, a financial manager, has loved good food all her life. And she has had a weight problem since she was a teenager. "I'd go on diets, lose a little weight, gain it back, lose it again. But about four years ago I gained a lot—over fifty pounds. Well, that was too much. I knew I should exercise, but I kept putting it off until I found something I enjoyed—aerobic dance. It's absolutely for me. I think it fits my hidden fantasy of being a dancer."

Through exercise alone, Juanita managed to lose about 25 pounds in 3 years. Then she heard about the Setpoint Diet. "That made a lot of sense to me," she says. "Maybe it's my affinity with numbers. Since I started Setpoint three months ago, I've lost twenty-three pounds. The exercise is still the most important thing, though. I try to not let anything interfere with it. It's my time. Not only does exercise make me feel good; I feel bad when I'm not exercising. It's like an addiction with me now. I feel deprived if I don't get to do it."

Aerobic dance may not be for you. But the point here is one that I cannot stress too strongly: Exercise makes you feel good. Once your body gets used to it, it begins to miss that feeling if you skip a day or two. Once you find the activity or activities that are "for you," as aerobic dance is for Juanita, you will find it is harder to skip your exercise session than it was at the beginning to make yourself get out and exercise in the first place.

I don't blame you if you are skeptical. And I know that it can be hard to think about beginning a program you will keep up your whole life. I know from personal experience that it's a lot easier *not to* exercise than *to* exercise. But whenever I stop exercising for any reason, I gain weight immediately—it seems like overnight. Even

more, I miss the energy and feeling of aliveness that comes
only from regular exercise.

## A Special Note for Women

It has been my observation that it is sometimes more
difficult for a woman to begin an exercise program than
for a man. Most men, after all, played sports from the
time they were young boys, and this is generally not the
case for women—particularly women over the age of 40
who were taught most of their lives that physical activity
is somehow "unladylike." Furthermore, you may be
reluctant to engage in any activities where you will have
to display a less-than-perfect body.

I can sympathize with your feelings, and I know too
that when you are overweight it is often difficult, say, to
get yourself out in the park walking, imagining that everyone is staring at you.

I want to reassure you that thousands of women, probably many of them in much poorer condition than you
are, have been able to start and stick with a regular program of moderate exercise. They have received not only
all the benefits we've talked about but also a tremendous
sense of self-esteem from knowing that they are doing
something special for themselves. Because it can be difficult, especially at the beginning, to stick with such a
program, read the tips in chapter 6 for ways to keep at it
until it becomes a natural part of your life.

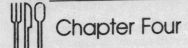

# Chapter Four

# Balance, Variety, Moderation

As you will soon see, the Setpoint Diet will be the easiest-to-follow diet you have ever gone on in your life—for the first time, your body will be working with you as you lose weight. Also, because the diet offers you such a variety and so much good food, you will never feel deprived or as if you are on a diet, even though you will be losing weight. Furthermore, all the details of calorie-counting and worrying about the proper nutrients are taken care of for you.

The cornerstones of the diet are balance, variety, and moderation. *Balance* means a balanced set of nutrients from all the basic food groups. *Variety* means you can choose from a wide variety of foods, including all of your favorites—even such things as candy and alcohol—that are forbidden on most diets. And *moderation* ensures that you learn to control the size of food portions that you eat.

Following this plan can change the way you eat—and think about eating—for a lifetime. The Setpoint plan has been tested on scores of volunteers, many of whom had been on other diets over the years without success, and they have been nearly unanimously enthusiastic about its benefits and the ease with which it can be maintained. Here is what a few of them have said:

"This was the only diet that I was able to eat candy bars and sweet rolls on and still lose weight: 25½ pounds in twelve weeks." (Richard Lesiak)

"Setpoint is terrific! It's the most effective program that I've tried. It is easy to stay on and very forgiving if you eat a little too much from time to time. I can only say why didn't I know about this years ago!" (Chuck Roberts, who lost 68 pounds)

"The diet teaches one how to eat properly and in what proportions. It allows you to 'cheat' every day. The diet is so liberal, it allows you to lead a normal life while dieting with little restriction. The best part is, this is how you will eat even after you quit dieting." (Jill M. Sweeney)

"I have tried every diet to come out in an effort to lose weight, but this plan has been the easiest to follow. I never felt denied. . . . As a matter of fact, I had a hard time eating all the food on the plan." (Sharon Kerkman)

This sort of enthusiasm is reflected by nearly everyone who has given the diet a fair chance. In this chapter I will explain how the Setpoint Diet works and, in the next two chapters, will give you specific instructions and guidelines for following the two parts of the plan.

Remember: Calorie reduction alone will *not* lower your setpoint; only the Setpoint exercise plan can do that. For best results you must combine both parts for a lifetime of slim, healthy living.

## Who Should Not Go on the Setpoint Diet

Although this is an extremely well-balanced, nourishing diet, the Setpoint Diet is not for everyone. Children, for example, should never go on a reduced-calorie diet without a doctor's supervision. Neither should pregnant or lactating women, or anyone with a serious chronic illness. Adolescents, who have different needs, can use a modified version of the Setpoint Diet. (See chapter 9.) If you require a special dietary regimen or have a medical history that suggests that exercise may not be advisable, contact your physician before deciding whether to follow the Setpoint Diet.

# Balance: The Setpoint Diet Food Groups

One reason the Setpoint Diet is different from many other weight-loss plans is that it includes all the foods needed in a healthy diet. Provided that you eat a variety of foods from each group and you eat the number of portions specified, you needn't worry about whether you are getting enough protein or vitamins or minerals; that is all taken care of for you. Here is how it works.

All foods fall into five basic Setpoint food groups, plus two Bonus groups and a Freebie group. The Bonus groups include all those items forbidden on most diets, such as gravy, butter, cookies, even alcohol. Depending upon your personal diet goals, you will have from two to four portions from each of the basic groups every day, plus a number of Bonus group treats.

The groupings are as follows: (1) Breads/Cereals/Starchy Foods; (2) Fruits; (3) Milk/Dairy Products; (4) Meat/Poultry/Fish; (5) Vegetables; and Bonus groups A and B and the Freebie group.

Servings from these groups may be combined in any way that you want throughout the day. In the next section of the book you will find simple daily menus to choose from—but you can modify them to suit yourself. For most people it is probably easiest and most comfortable to eat three meals a day, supplemented with snacks. But if another combination of meals fits your needs better, the Setpoint Diet is flexible enough to accommodate it. However, you must eat the number of portions specified for each food group—it is vital to get the proper nutrition while you diet.

In the following chapters are sample charts that will help people to keep track of each food group every day. Several volunteers who have been on the diet have reported that there is so much food available it is often difficult to eat all the food specified for daily consumption.

## Variety: Choosing within the Groups

The Setpoint Diet emphasizes variety, both among the food groups and within them (thus, in the Breads/Cereals/Starchy Foods group, you are encouraged to choose different foods: a bran muffin at one meal, pasta at another, and perhaps a starchy vegetable at a third). Don't eat the same foods all the time!

Variety is especially important psychologically as well as for your physical health: knowing that you can have a piece of cake and still stay on your diet can be just the incentive you need to keep going and continue losing weight until you have reached your goal.

## Moderation: Forget about Calories—Use Portion Control

You have probably been on a number of calorie-counting diets at one time or another, and you know the agony of deciding whether you can afford to eat another mouthful of pudding or another potato chip. The Setpoint Diet makes this a worry of the past.

Instead of calorie-counting, the Setpoint Diet relies on portion control; portion sizes are prescribed, and the number of portions you have each day depends on how much weight you want to lose. Most people like to measure or weigh the food initially to determine if it is the right amount. After they are on the diet for a few days they learn approximate weights and measures, so portion control becomes easier.

Thus, all you have to do is eat the correct number of portions in servings of the correct size. Each portion allowed for any item in one food group is roughly equivalent calorically to any other item in that group. In the Breads/Cereals/Starchy Foods group, for example, ½ bagel counts as one portion; so does one tortilla, and so does ½ large ear of corn. Some foods, of course, are combinations from different groups (one cup of chicken chow mein is equal to one Meat/Poultry/Fish and two Vegetables portions).

## Why You Needn't Give Up Your Favorite Food and Drink

One reason that other diets are so difficult to stick with, apart from their failure to work, is that we inevitably feel deprived while following them. Food is important to us not only for nutrition but also for psychological and social reasons. Eating food figures prominently in our family lives and in our social lives. And this is to be expected, since everyone has favorite foods. Often these are rich foods, such as pie, or ethnic delights, such as strudel. On traditional diets these foods are not allowed—a rule that is self-defeating. Why should we deny ourselves the enjoyment of foods that are important in our lives?

"But eating sweet and fatty foods isn't healthy," some experts might say. My answer to that is that all foods *can* and *should* be part of a balanced diet—it's deprivation that isn't healthy!

The key to the success of this diet plan is moderation. A diet of bean sprouts and wheat germ would be unhealthy if that were all that you ever ate.

Likewise, most diets forbid alcoholic drinks. As you will see in the next section, moderate amounts of beer and wine—even an occasional cocktail—are allowed on the Setpoint Diet. Again, the idea is moderation.

The Setpoint Diet is designed to be a plan you can follow for a lifetime: not just while you're losing weight but later, too—when you're trying to keep the lost weight off. You should continue to observe the Setpoint principles—balance, variety, and moderation—for the rest of your life, though you will be able to eat more food portions than when you were losing weight. No diet that forces you to eliminate favorite foods and drink forever is very realistic, because you probably won't stay on it.

## Your Personal Goals— Individualization

Unlike many traditional calorie-controlled diets, the Setpoint Diet allows you to choose the calorie level that's right for you. A standard 1500- or 1200-calorie diet for everyone simply makes no sense, given the wide variation in people's needs. The Setpoint Diet is individualized to best help you meet your own weight-loss goals in the shortest period of time while you lose weight gradually and safely.

Choosing your own plan is easy—it is based on your own weight goal. In the next chapter I will explain how to choose your own individual plan.

## Vitamin Supplements—Yes or No?

Most Americans who eat a healthy, balanced diet receive all the micronutrients—vitamins and minerals—that they need through the food they are eating. However, there is a danger that people who go on low-calorie diets, especially those below 1200 calories a day, might not receive all the nutrients that they need for optimum health.

If you are on Setpoint's 1200-calorie diet plan, then, it may be a good idea, though it's by no means essential, to take a multiple vitamin and mineral supplement every day, especially one containing vitamin B6, magnesium, iron (especially for females), calcium, and zinc—nutrients often lacking in the American diet. But beware of "megavitamin" products offering more than 100 percent of the U.S. Recommended Daily Allowance; excess amounts of some vitamins can accumulate to dangerous levels in the body.

## Why the Setpoint Diet Does What Other Diets Can't

I want to reiterate that calorie reduction alone cannot lower your Setpoint. Only daily exercise can do that. But the Setpoint Diet—which combines portion control with moderate daily exercise—can do many things that other diets can't do.

It is easy to follow in restaurants and other people's homes. It does allow you to have sweets—every day, if you wish—or a couple of beers. And it also makes you aware of your own eating habits and retrains you to eat more nutritiously. By including all the different food groups, you learn to eat the most healthful mix of foods every day. By practicing portion control, you learn to eat in moderation. And by emphasizing a wide variety of foods that may be eaten throughout the day, you learn to eat in such a way that you are never ravenous and thus tempted to binge.

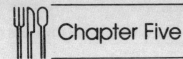 **Chapter Five**

# How to Use the Diet

Now that you understand the principles behind the Setpoint Diet, it is time to get started! Please read through this chapter, paying particular attention to the charts, to get an idea of what you will need to do to follow the plan.

## Step One: Find Your Desirable Weight.

On p. 34 is a chart showing desirable weights, based on lowest mortality, for adults from ages 25 to 59. I suggest that you use the chart as a guide only, however; the best weight for you depends on a number of factors, including your age and your build.

If you were lean when you were about 20 years old, your weight at that time can provide a reasonable goal. If you have never been slim in your adult life, choose an approximate weight based on the chart; as you lose, you can adjust your goal if necessary. In any case, don't choose an unrealistic weight goal: If you have big bones you're *never* going to look skinny!

# Step Two: Set a Realistic Weight-Loss Schedule.

This step is optional, but it may provide extra motivation to keep you going in the early days. After you have chosen your weight-loss goal (say, 20 pounds), target the date that you expect to reach it. Remember that you didn't put those pounds on overnight, so you can't expect to lose them overnight.

For maximum effectiveness and safety, you should plan to lose weight at the safe and healthy rate of 1 to 3 pounds per week. The more weight you have to lose, the more quickly you will probably lose, especially at the beginning. Anything more than 3 or so pounds per week, however, is too fast a loss—that usually signifies the loss of body fluid or muscle mass rather than fat.

# Step Three: Start Your Exercise Program.

Remember that portion control alone will not lower your setpoint—only an exercise plan can do that. Don't put off your exercise plan. Begin it at the same time you begin portion control. In the next chapter are specific instructions to help you determine the best combination of activities for your needs.

# Step Four: Choose Your Personalized Eating Plan.

The Setpoint Diet allows you to choose from five eating plans that reflect different calorie intake levels: 1200, 1500, 1800, 2100, and 2400.

To decide which plan you should follow, first calculate your daily calorie needs according to the following formula:

Desired weight × 10 = daily calories needed to *lose* weight.

For example, if you weigh 146 pounds but you want to weigh 127 pounds, multiply your desired weight, 127 pounds, by 10. The result is 1270 calories a day.

Next choose the eating plan closest to the calorie level

## Weight Chart

| Height (ft, In) | Men Small Frame | Medium Frame | Large Frame | Women Small Frame | Medium Frame | Large Frame |
|---|---|---|---|---|---|---|
| 4'10" | | | | 102-111 | 109-121 | 118-131 |
| 4'11" | | | | 103-113 | 111-123 | 120-134 |
| 5'0" | | | | 104-115 | 113-126 | 122-137 |
| 5'1" | | | | 106-118 | 115-129 | 125-140 |
| 5'2" | 128-134 | 131-141 | 138-150 | 108-121 | 118-132 | 128-143 |
| 5'3" | 130-136 | 133-143 | 140-153 | 111-124 | 121-135 | 131-147 |
| 5'4" | 132-138 | 135-145 | 142-156 | 114-127 | 124-138 | 134-151 |
| 5'5" | 134-140 | 137-148 | 144-160 | 117-130 | 127-141 | 137-155 |
| 5'6" | 136-142 | 139-151 | 146-164 | 120-133 | 130-144 | 140-159 |
| 5'7" | 138-145 | 142-154 | 149-168 | 123-136 | 133-147 | 143-163 |
| 5'8" | 140-148 | 145-157 | 152-172 | 126-139 | 136-150 | 146-167 |
| 5'9" | 142-151 | 148-160 | 155-176 | 129-142 | 139-153 | 149-170 |
| 5'10" | 144-154 | 151-163 | 158-180 | 132-145 | 142-156 | 152-173 |
| 5'11" | 146-157 | 154-166 | 161-184 | 135-148 | 145-159 | 155-176 |
| 6'0" | 149-160 | 157-170 | 164-188 | 138-151 | 148-162 | 158-179 |
| 6'1" | 152-164 | 160-174 | 168-192 | | | |
| 6'2" | 155-168 | 164-178 | 172-197 | | | |
| 6'3" | 158-172 | 167-182 | 176-202 | | | |
| 6'4" | 162-176 | 171-187 | 181-207 | | | |

Weights at ages 25–59 based on lowest mortality. Weight in pounds according to frame (in indoor clothing weighing 5 lbs. for men, 3 lbs. for women; height in shoes with 1-in. heels).

Source: 1983 Metropolitan Height and Weight Tables, Metropolitan Life Insurance Company.

you need. In the example above, where your daily calorie need was 1270 calories, you should choose the 1200-calorie diet plan. If your daily calorie need were 1700 calories, you would choose the 1800-calorie plan.

In some cases, the daily calorie need will fall midway between two of the plans (for example, 1650 calories). In that case, choose the lower-calorie plan and begin the diet. If you find that you are losing weight too quickly or that you feel weak and hungry, switch to the next higher-calorie plan. The results may come a little more slowly, but that will be better for you long-term.

If your calculation indicates fewer than 1200 calories are needed, choose the 1200-calorie diet anyway. As long as you exercise faithfully you will probably lose weight on this plan. It can be dangerous to go on a diet of fewer than 1200 calories except under a doctor's supervision; any diet that is so severely restricted in calories is almost certain to be deficient in important nutrients as well.

Remember that the Setpoint Diet is based on the nutritional needs of the average healthy adult. It is not designed for use by those with special dietary needs, such as children and pregnant or lactating women. Also, if you are extremely overweight (twice or more ideal body weight), you should diet only under a doctor's supervision. For information on Setpoint for adolescents and older people, see chapters 9 and 10.

## Step Five: Start the Portion Control Program.

Familiarize yourself with the basic food groups. You'll be eating a specified number of portions from each group every day. Portions for the foods in each group are roughly equivalent calorically. The groups are as follows:

*Breads/Cereals/Starchy Foods* (p. 36), which includes breads, pasta, and starchy vegetables like corn, beans, and potatoes.
*Fruits* (p. 37), including fruit juices.

*Milk/Dairy Products* (p. 38), including cheeses and ice cream.

*Meat/Poultry/Fish* (p. 39), which also includes eggs and tofu (soybean curd).

*Vegetables* (p. 40), comprising all vegetables except those that are high in starch.

## Breads/Cereals/ Starchy Foods

| | |
|---|---|
| ½ | Bagel, Matzoh |
| 1 small | Biscuit |
| 1 slice | Bread |
| 2 medium | Bread Sticks, plain |
| ¼ cup | Bread Crumbs, dry |
| 2 tbsp | Flour |
| 2 squares | Graham Crackers |
| ½ | Roll—Hard, Hamburger, Hot Dog |
| 1 small | Roll—Dinner, Crescent |
| ½ | Muffin—Blueberry, Bran Corn, English, Plain |
| ½ large | Pita Bread |
| 3 cups popped | Popcorn |
| 10 | Pretzel Rings, single |
| 6 | Saltines or other small crackers |
| 4 pieces | Melba Toast |
| 1 | Tortilla, 6 inch |
| 2 | Zwieback |
| ½ cup cooked | Oatmeal, Grits, Farina, Cream of Rice, Whole Wheat Cereal |
| ½ cup | Ready–to–Eat Cereals except Granola types (See B Bonus Foods) |
| ¼ cup | Beans—Baked, Garbanzo |
| ½ cup cooked | Pasta—Macaroni, Spaghetti, Noodles |
| ½ medium | Potato—baked, boiled |
| ½ cup | Potato, mashed |
| ⅓ cup cooked | Rice |
| ¼ cup | Sweet Potato or Yam |
| ⅓ cup | Corn, Black-Eyed Peas, Lentils, Lima Beans |
| ½ cup | Peas, Peas & Carrots, Winter Squash |
| ½ large ear | Corn on the Cob |

## Fruits

|  | **Fresh, canned, or frozen unsweetened fruits** |
|---|---|
| 1 small | Apple |
| ½ medium | Apple |
| ⅓ cup | Apple Juice |
| ½ cup | Applesauce |
| ½ cup | Apricot halves |
| ⅓ cup | Apricot Nectar |
| 2 medium | Apricots |
| ⅛ | Avocado |
| ½ small | Banana |
| ½ cup | Blueberries |
| ¼ | Cantaloupe |
| 10 | Cherries |
| ½ cup | Citrus sections |
| ⅓ cup | Cranberry Juice |
| 2 | Dates, Prunes |
| 1 | Fig, dried or fresh |
| ½ cup | Fruit Cocktail |
| ⅓ cup | Grape Juice |
| ½ small | Grapefruit |
| ½ cup | Grapefruit Juice |
| 12 | Grapes |
| 1/10 | Honeydew Melon |
| 1 small | Nectarine |
| ½ cup | Mandarin Oranges |
| 1 small | Orange |
| ⅓ cup | Orange Juice |
| 1 medium | Peach |
| ½ cup | Peach halves or slices |
| ½ medium | Pear |
| ½ cup | Pear halves or slices |
| ½ cup | Pineapple Chunks |
| ⅓ cup | Pineapple Juice |
| 2 small | Plums |
| ¼ cup | Prune Juice |
| 2 tbsp | Raisins |
| ¾ cup | Strawberries |
| 1 medium | Tangerine |
| 1 cup | Watermelon |

## Milk/Dairy Products

| | | |
|---|---|---|
| **1 cup** | Buttermilk | |
| **1 cup** | 1% Low-fat Milk | |
| **1 cup** | Skim Milk | |
| **1 oz** | Swiss Cheese | |
| **1½ oz** | Mozzarella Cheese, part skim | |
| **¼ cup** | Parmesan or Romano Cheese, grated | |
| **⅓ cup** | Ricotta Cheese, part skim | |

| | **Additional Choices** | **Portion Equivalents** |
|---|---|---|
| **1 cup** | Whole Milk | 1 Milk and 1 A Bonus |
| **1 cup** | 2% Low-fat Milk | 1 Milk and ½ A Bonus |
| **1 cup** | Low-fat Chocolate Milk | 1 Milk and 1 A Bonus |
| **1 cup** | Hot Cocoa, whole milk | 1 Milk and 2 A Bonus |
| **1 cup** | Low-fat or whole Yogurt, plain | 1 Milk and ½ A Bonus |
| **1 cup** | Low-fat Yogurt, flavored | 1 Milk and 1½ A Bonus |
| **1 cup** | Low-fat Yogurt, fruited | 1 Milk and 2 A Bonus |
| **1½ oz** | Blue Cheese | 1 Milk and 1 A Bonus |
| **2½ oz** | Camembert Cheese | 1 Milk and 2 A Bonus |
| **1½ oz** | Cheddar Cheese | 1 Milk and 1 A Bonus |
| **2 oz** | Cheese Spread | 1 Milk and 1 A Bonus |
| **1 cup** | Cottage Cheese, 1% fat | 1 Milk and 1 A Bonus |
| **1 cup** | Cottage Cheese, creamed | 1 Milk and 2 A Bonus |
| **2 oz** | Feta Cheese | 1 Milk and 1 A Bonus |
| **1½ oz** | Gouda Cheese | 1 Milk and 1 A Bonus |
| **1¼ oz** | Monterey Cheese | 1 Milk and ½ A Bonus |
| **2 oz** | Mozzarella Cheese, whole milk | 1 Milk and 1 A Bonus |
| **1¼ oz** | Muenster Cheese | 1 Milk and ½ A Bonus |
| **1½ oz** | Port du Salut Cheese | 1 Milk and 1 A Bonus |
| **1½ oz** | Process American Cheese | 1 Milk and 1 A Bonus |
| **1¼ oz** | Provolone Cheese | 1 Milk and ½ A Bonus |
| **¾ cup** | Ice Cream or Sherbet | ½ Milk and 2½ A Bonus |
| **1 cup** | Ice Milk | ½ Milk and 2 A Bonus |

Meat/Poultry/Fish

**Cooked with visible fat removed—
broiled, roasted, or baked**

| | |
|---|---|
| **2 oz** | Beef—Very lean Chuck or Ground Beef, Corned Beef, Flank Steak, Rib Eye, Round, Rump, Sirloin |
| **2 oz** | Chicken/Turkey—Dark meat, no skin |
| **3 oz** | Chicken/Turkey—White meat, no skin |
| **4 oz** | Crab, Lobster |
| **2 oz** | Fish—Fatty—Herring, Mackerel |
| **3 oz** | Fish—Medium fat—Bluefish, Salmon, Swordfish |
| **4 oz** | Fish—Lowfat—Cod, Flounder, Haddock, Halibut, Sole |
| **2 oz** | Ham, Canadian Bacon, Chopped Ham, Ham & Cheese Loaf |
| **4 oz** | 95% Fat-Free Ham |
| **2 oz** | Lamb—Leg, Loin Roast or Chops, Shoulder |
| **2 oz** | Liver, Heart, Kidney, Sweetbreads |
| **2 oz** | Meatloaf, Meatballs |
| **2 oz** | Pork—Loin, Picnic, Boston Butt |
| **2 oz** | Veal—Cutlets, Leg, Loin, Rib, Shank |
| **3 oz** | 90% Fat-Free Luncheon Meat |
| **3 slices** | Chicken or Turkey Roll |
| **10 medium** | Clams, Scallops, Oysters, Mussels |
| **2** | Eggs |
| **2 slices** | Salami—Beef, Pork, Turkey |
| **5 medium** | Sardines—canned, drained |
| **10 large** | Shrimp |
| **1 piece** | Tofu—(soybean curd) 2½ in. x 2½ in. x 2 in. |
| **½ cup** | Tuna—canned in water or oil, drained |

| | **Additional Choices** | **Portion Equivalents** |
|---|---|---|
| **4 strips** | Bacon | ½ Meat and 2 A Bonus |
| **2 slices** | Bologna | 1 Meat and 1 A Bonus |
| **1 link** | Bratwurst | 1 Meat and 2 A Bonus |
| **3 slices** | Braunschweiger | 1 Meat and 1 A Bonus |
| **4 links** | Breakfast Sausage | 1 Meat and 1½ A Bonus |
| **2 oz** | Deviled Ham | 1 Meat and 1 A Bonus |
| **1 medium** | Frank or Wiener | 1 Meat and 1 A Bonus |
| **2 oz** | Ground Beef, regular | 1 Meat and ½ A Bonus |
| **6 slices** | Hard Salami | 1 Meat and 2 A Bonus |

| | | |
|---|---|---|
| **1 link** | Italian Sausage | 1 Meat and 1½ A Bonus |
| **1 link** | Knockwurst | 1 Meat and 1½ A Bonus |
| **2 slices** | Luncheon Meat | 1 Meat and ½ A Bonus |
| **2 patties** | Pork Sausage | 1 Meat and 1½ A Bonus |
| **2 oz** | Spare Ribs, lean | 1 Meat and 1½ A Bonus |

## Vegetables

**½ cup raw or cooked**
Artichoke Hearts
Asparagus
Bean Sprouts
Beets
Broccoli
Brussels Sprouts
Carrots
Collard Greens
Eggplant
Green Beans
Kale
Mustard Greens
Onions
Sauerkraut
Spinach, cooked
Tomato Juice
Tomatoes
Turnip
Turnip Greens
Vegetable Juice Cocktail
Wax Beans

**⅓ cup**
Tomato Sauce

**1 cup raw or cooked**
Beet Greens
Cabbage
Cauliflower
Celery
Cucumber
Green or Red Pepper
Mushrooms

                    Radishes
                    Summer Squash
                    Zucchini Squash

    **2 cups raw**  Endive
                    Lettuce
                    Spinach
                    Watercress

                    **See Breads/Cereals/Starchy
                    Foods list for
                    starchy vegetables**


    You will also need to familiarize yourself with the Bonus
groups, Freebies, and Combination Foods. The A and B
Bonus groups are found on pages 42–43. These lists contain most high-calorie as well as snack foods. On the A
list you will find such fatty foods as butter, mayonnaise,
sauces, dressings, and sour cream that in small amounts
add palatability and a feeling of "richness" to a meal. On
the A and B lists are such snack foods as nuts and potato
chips, as well as desserts and alcoholic beverages. The
Bonus groups are intended to give the diet flexibility. You
can either enjoy the Bonus Foods or convert Bonus portions to extra portions of food from the other groups. (See
"Or Substitute" sections of the Bonus lists.)
    Freebies (p. 44). This list includes "free," no- or low-
calorie foods, such as coffee, tea, seasonings, and con-
diments. Note that some of the Freebies are limited to
two portions per day.
    Some combination foods—those that contain ingre-
dients from more than one food group—are found on page
44.

## A Bonus Foods

| | |
|---|---|
| 2 tsp | Butter, Margarine |
| 2 tsp | Vegetable Oil |
| 2 tsp | Mayonnaise |
| 2 tbsp | Reduced-Calorie Mayonaise |
| 2 tsp | Salad Dressing, regular |
| 2 tbsp | Coffee Whitener, liquid |
| 2 tbsp | Coffee Whitener, powdered |
| 1 tbsp | Cream, light or heavy |
| 2 tbsp | Brie Cheese |
| 1 tbsp | Cream Cheese |
| 2 tbsp | Half & Half |
| 2 tbsp | Sour Cream |
| 2 tbsp | Whipped Cream, unsweetened |
| 3 tbsp | Whipped Topping, dairy or nondairy |
| 2 tbsp | Sauce—cheese, cream |
| 2 tbsp | Gravy |
| 3 tbsp | Sweet & Sour Sauce |
| ⅓ cup | Barbecue Sauce |
| 2 tbsp | Seasoned Coating Mix |
| 2 small | Sweet Gherkin Pickles |
| 2 tbsp | Coconut shredded |
| 10 | Olives |
| 10 | Almonds |
| 4 large | Cashews |
| 10 large | Peanuts |
| 2 large | Pecans, whole |
| 2 medium | Walnuts, whole |
| 1 tbsp | Sunflower Seeds |
| 1 medium | Cookie |
| ½ cup | Fruit-flavored Gelatin |
| 1 small | Sugar-type Cone for Ice Cream |
| 1 bar | Frozen Pudding on a stick, uncoated |
| 6 large | Jelly Beans |
| 4 tsp | Jelly, Jam |
| 4 tsp | Sugar, white or brown |
| 1 tbsp | Honey or Syrup |
| 1 tbsp | Dessert Topping—Butterscotch, Hot Fudge, Lemon, etc. |
| 6 fl oz | Breakfast or Soft Drinks, noncarbonated |
| 6 fl oz | International Flavored Coffee |
| 8 fl oz | Beer, light |
| ½ fl oz | Brandies, Cordials |
| 1 fl oz | Gin, Rum Vodka, Whiskey |

| 3 fl oz | Wine or Sherry, dry |
| 4 fl oz | Wine, light |

**Or Substitute:**

| 1 portion | Breads/Cereals/Starchy Foods |
| 2 portions | Fruits |
| ½ portion | Milk/Dairy products |
| 3 portions | Vegetables |
| ½ portion | Meat/Poultry/Fish |

## B Bonus Foods

| ⅛ | Angel Food Cake |
| ½ in. slice | Applesauce or Carrot Cake |
| 1 medium | Brownie |
| 1½ oz | Candy Bar, Fudge |
| 1/12 | Cheesecake |
| 3 tbsp | Chocolate Chips |
| 1 medium | Cinnamon Roll |
| ⅓ cup | Cranberry Sauce |
| 1 medium | Croissant |
| 1 medium | Cupcake with icing |
| ⅛ | Danish Ring, plain |
| 1 medium | Doughnut |
| ⅛ | Gingerbread Cake, unfrosted |
| ⅓ cup | Granola Cereal |
| ¾ cup | Italian Ice |
| 1/16 | Layer Cake with icing |
| 2 tbsp | Peanut Butter |
| 1/12 | Pie—Chiffon, Cream, Custard, Fruit |
| 15 | Potato Chips |
| ¾ in. slice | Pound Cake, plain |
| ½ in. slice | Quick Breads—Banana, Cranberry, Date Nut, Pumpkin |
| 1 individual | Tart of Pastry Shell |
| 1¼ oz | Tortilla or Corn Chips |
| 12 fl oz | Soft Drinks, carbonated |
| 12 fl oz | Beer or Ale |
| 4 fl oz | Wine or Sherry, sweet |

**Or Substitute**

| 3 portions | Breads/Cereals/Starchy Foods |
| 4 portions | Fruits |
| 2 portions | Milk/Dairy Products |
| 1½ portions | Meat/Poultry/Fish |
| 3 portions | A Bonus Foods |

Freebies

Coffee, black
Tea, plain
Bouillon
Diet/Sugar-Free Soft Drinks
Club Soda
Water
Artificial Sweetener
Mustard
Lemon or Lime Juice
Pimiento
Soy Sauce, Vinegar
Salt & Pepper
Herbs—Basil, Bay Leaf, Dill,
    Oregano, Parsley, etc.
Spices—Chili, Cloves,
    Cinnamon, Curry, Sage, etc.

**Limit to two portions
per day:**

|          |                              |
|----------|------------------------------|
| 1        | Dill Pickle                  |
| 4 slices | Bread 'n Butter Pickles      |
| 1 tbsp   | Catsup, Cocktail Sauce       |
| 1 tbsp   | Horseradish                  |
| 1 tbsp   | Low-Calorie Salad Dressing   |
| 2 tsp    | Relish, sweet                |
| ½ cup    | Low-Calorie Gelatin          |
| 2 tbsp   | Reduced-Calorie Whipped Topping |
| ¼ cup    | Taco Sauce                   |
| 1 small  | Wafer-type Cone for Ice Cream |

## Combination Foods

|          |                        | **Portion Equivalents**                     |
|----------|------------------------|---------------------------------------------|
| 3 slices | French Toast           | 3 Bread, ½ Meat, and 1 A Bonus              |
| 4 medium | Pancakes               | 2 Bread, ½ Meat, and ½ A Bonus              |
| 3 small  | Waffles                | 2 Bread, ½ Meat, and 1 A Bonus              |
| 1        | Burrito, Beef and Bean | 2 Bread, ½ Meat, and 1 A Bonus              |
| 1 cup    | Chicken Chow Mein      | 1 meat and 2 Veg                            |
| 1 cup    | Chili with Beans       | 2 Bread, 1 Meat, 1 Veg and ½ A Bonus        |

| 3 in. x 3 in. x 3 in. | Lasagna | 1 Bread, 1 Meat, 2 Veg, 2 Milk, and 1 A Bonus |
|---|---|---|
| 1 cup | Macaroni and Cheese | 2 Bread, ½ Milk, and a A Bonus |
| ⅙ large pie | Pizza, Cheese | 1 Bread, 1 Veg, ½ Milk, and 1 A Bonus |
| ⅙ pie | Quiche, plain | 1 Bread, ½ Meat, 1 Milk, and 1 A Bonus |
| 2 | Tacos, Beef or Chicken | 2 Bread, 1½ Meat, 1 Veg, ½ Milk, and ½ A Bonus |
| ½ cup | Bread Stuffing | 1½ Bread and 1 A Bonus |
| 10 medium | French Fries | 1 Bread, and 1½ A Bonus |
| ½ cup | Seasoned Rice Mixes | 1½ Bread, and ½ A Bonus |
| ½ cup | Cole Slaw | ½ Veg and 1 A Bonus |
| ½ cup | Macaroni or Potato Salad | 1 Bread and 1 A Bonus |
| ½ cup | Custard, baked | ½ Meat, ½ Milk, and ½ A Bonus |
| ½ cup | Fruit, canned, sweetened | 1 Fruit and 1 A Bonus |
| ½ cup | Pudding, regular | ½ Milk and 2 A Bonus |
| ½ cup | Pudding, reduced-calorie | ½ Milk and ½ A Bonus |

**Soups, prepared with water**

| 8 fl oz | Chicken Noodle | ½ Bread and ½ A Bonus |
|---|---|---|
| 7½ fl oz | Chunky Beef | 1 Bread, ½ Meat, and 1 Veg |
| 8 fl oz | Clam Chowder, Manhattan | 1 Bread |
| 8 fl oz | Cream of Mushroom | ½ Bread and 1½ A Bonus |
| 8 fl oz | Split Pea with Ham | 1 Bread, ½ Meat, and ½ A Bonus |
| 8 fl oz | Tomato | 1 Bread and ½ Veg |
| 8 fl oz | Vegetable | 1 Bread and ½ Veg |

Look at the Setpoint portion chart for adults below. This tells you the number of portions allowed from each Setpoint Diet food group for each calorie level.

| The Setpoint Diet for Adults: Portions per Day | | | | | |
|---|---|---|---|---|---|
| | *CALORIES* | | | | |
| | *1200* | *1500* | *1800* | *2100* | *2400* |
| | *Portions per Day* | | | | |
| *Breads/Cereals/ Starchy Foods* | 4 | 4 | 4 | 4 | 4 |
| *Fruits* | 3 | 3 | 3 | 3 | 3 |
| *Milk/Dairy Products* | 2 | 2 | 2 | 2 | 2 |
| *Meat/Poultry/ Fish* | 2 | 2 | 2 | 2 | 2 |
| *Vegetables* | 3 | 3 | 3 | 3 | 3 |
| *A Bonus* | 2 | 4 | 5 | 7 | 9 |
| *B Bonus* | 1 | 2 | 3 | 4 | 5 |

To ensure balanced nutrition, you must eat all portions specified for each of the five main groups, combined in any way you wish. For example, for lunch you might have a turkey sandwich with mayo (2 Breads/Cereals/Starchy Foods, 1 Meat/Poultry/Fish, 1 A Bonus), an apple (1 Fruits), and a glass of tea (a freebie). Whatever you have for lunch, of course, must be considered and planned in the context of your total food intake for the day.

Eat only the amount of food listed per portion (2 oz, 1 cup, etc.). Measure or weigh your foods—at least until you are familiar with the portion sizes. (Most Setpointers report that this becomes automatic within a few days or weeks at most.) Remember: cooked foods should be measured or weighed after cooking.

Keep a daily record of the portions you eat. On pages 48–52 are sample portion-control records for each of the five calorie levels for adults. Make several copies and

carry one with you each day. Fill in all portions you consume at each meal and snack, and total them at the end
of the day to be certain that you have not gone over or
under your portion allowance for any group. Simple check
marks will do if you don't want a record of just what
you've eaten.

# A Note for Calorie Counters

If you are like some chronic dieters, you may feel
uncomfortable with "portions"; you may prefer calorie-
counting. The Setpoint Diet is, in fact, calorie-controlled,
and for most people it is easier to count a few portions a
day rather than calculate hundreds of calories. But if you
feel more comfortable knowing the calorie content of all
foods you eat, refer to the following chart.

## Setpoint Calorie Chart

This table gives you calorie ranges for the Setpoint
food groups

| | Calories per Portion |
| --- | --- |
| Breads/Cereals/Starchy Foods | 60–80 |
| Fruits | 30–50 |
| Milk/Dairy Products | 85–110 |
| Meat/Poultry/Fish | 110–150 |
| Vegetables | 15–30 |
| A Bonus | 40–90 |
| B Bonus | 150–220 |
| Freebies | Fewer than 15 |

# 1200 Calorie Portion Checklist for Adults

Date _____

| Breads/Cereals/ Starchy Foods | Fruits | Milk/Dairy Products | Meat/Fish/ Poultry | Vegetables | A Bonus | B Bonus |
|---|---|---|---|---|---|---|
| | | | | | | |
| | | | | | | |
| | | | | | | |
| | | | | | | |

## 1500 Calorie Portion Checklist for Adults

Date _____

| Breads/Cereals/Starchy Foods | Fruits | Milk/Dairy Products | Meat/Fish/Poultry | Vegetables | A Bonus | B Bonus |
|---|---|---|---|---|---|---|
|  |  |  |  |  |  |  |
|  |  |  |  |  |  |  |
|  |  |  |  |  |  |  |

## 1800 Calorie Portion Checklist for Adults

Date _____

| Breads/Cereals/Starchy Foods | Fruits | Milk/Dairy Products | Meat/Fish/Poultry | Vegetables | A Bonus | B Bonus |
|---|---|---|---|---|---|---|
| | | | | | | |
| | | | | | | |
| | | | | | | |
| | | | | | | |

# 2100 Calorie Portion Checklist for Adults

Date _____

| Breads/Cereals/ Starchy Foods | Fruits | Milk/Dairy Products | Meat/Fish/ Poultry | Vegetables | A Bonus | B Bonus |
|---|---|---|---|---|---|---|
| | | | | | | |
| | | | | | | |
| | | | | | | |
| | | | | | | |
| | | | | | | |

# 2400 Calorie Portion Checklist for Adults

Date _____

| Breads/Cereals/Starchy Foods | Fruits | Milk/Dairy Products | Meat/Fish/Poultry | Vegetables | A Bonus | B Bonus |
|---|---|---|---|---|---|---|
|  |  |  |  |  |  |  |
|  |  |  |  |  |  |  |
|  |  |  |  |  |  |  |
|  |  |  |  |  |  |  |
|  |  |  |  |  |  |  |
|  |  |  |  |  |  |  |
|  |  |  |  |  |  |  |
|  |  |  |  |  |  |  |

# Enjoy Eating

And now you're ready to begin losing weight gradually and comfortably while enjoying good eating.

If one of your favorite foods isn't listed, count it as a food that is similar. Thus, ⅓ cup of black beans, which is similar to the starchy vegetables corn and lentils, would count as 1 Breads/Cereals/Starchy Foods portion. Or, if you know the number of calories contained in a given amount of the food (from the food label, for example), you can use the calorie chart on p. 47 to determine how much of that food would equal one portion. Many products now list calorie content on their labels.

# How to Figure Out Combination Foods

Combination foods—stews, casseroles, sandwiches— are all included in the Setpoint plan. On p. 54 there is a list of many of the most popular Combination Foods, giving portion information for each.

When preparing and eating combination foods that aren't on the list, you will need to determine your own portion information. Bear in mind that since Combination Foods contain foods from more than one of the Setpoint Diet food groups, each of these foods—including cooking oil—should be counted when you are calculating portion information. (Remember to record the various portions from the combination food on your daily food record.)

If you are not sure of all the ingredients in a combination food, refer to a recipe if possible. When dining out, don't be afraid to ask the waiter how a dish is prepared. You'll be surprised how easy it will become to estimate portions in a restaurant once you have some experience with weighing and measuring different foods at home. Don't be afraid to estimate—just rely on your experience and be as accurate as you can.

For more information on computing combination foods, see pages 54–56.

## Assessing Combination Foods

Here are five easy steps to determine how combination foods break down into portions from the various Setpoint food groups. The last two steps may not be needed unless you are computing portions for complex recipes.

1. Identify the Setpoint Diet food groups in the combination food, visually or by using the recipe.
2. Determine the number of Setpoint portions for each ingredient. (See food group lists, pp. 36–41 and the Setpoint Guide to Ingredients, p. 132.) If the ingredient does not appear on either list, estimate! Use information given for a comparable ingredient. And—for help with weights and measures—see the Measurement Conversion Table on p. 133.
3. Total the portions from each food group.
4. Round the total number of portions for each food group to the nearest half portion (1 $\frac{1}{12}$ portions = 1 portion; $\frac{2}{3}$ portion = $\frac{1}{2}$ portion). This is done for simplicity's sake, making it easier for you to keep track of the total number of portions you eat during the day from each group.
5. To determine how many Setpoint portions are in each serving of a dish, divide the total number of portions for each food group by the number of servings in the dish or recipe. (Again, round to the nearest half portion.)

To see how this works in practice, let's look at some examples.

Basic Cheeseburger   This is an easy food to visualize. Only the first three steps are necessary for determining portions:

1. A cheeseburger consists of beef, cheese, and a roll— these are found, respectively, in the following food groups: Meat/Poultry/Fish; Milk/Dairy Products; and Breads/Cereals/Starchy Foods.
2. and 3. If the cheeseburger has 3 oz cooked beef and ¾ oz American cheese, then:

   3 oz cooked beef = 1½ portions of Meat/Poultry/Fish;
   ¾ oz American cheese = ½ Milk/Dairy Products and ½ A Bonus; and
   1 hamburger roll = 2 Breads/Cereals/Starchy Foods.

Note: Remember to weigh the hamburger meat *after* cooking. If you're eating out, ask what the cooked weight is.

Now let's take a more complicated example.

Chicken Vegetable Casserole   This recipe, which serves three, consists of the following ingredients: 9 oz cooked light chicken; 3 tbsp butter; ½ cup diced celery; ⅓ cup sliced onion; ⅓ cup sliced green pepper; 3 tbsp enriched flour; 1½ cups chicken broth; 1 egg; 3 tbsp white wine; ⅔ cup cooked rice.

1. Identify the food groups. Chicken and eggs are in the Meat/Poultry/Fish group; butter and white wine are A Bonuses; celery, onion, and green pepper are all in the Vegetables group; and flour and rice are on the Breads/Cereals/Starchy Foods list.
2. Determine the number of Setpoint portions for each ingredient:

   9 oz cooked light chicken = 3 Meat/Poultry/Fish
   3 tbsp butter = 4½ A Bonus
   ½ cup celery ⎫
   ⅓ cup onion ⎬ = totals approx 1½ Vegetables
   ⅓ cup green pepper ⎭
   3 tbsp flour = approx 1 Breads/Cereals/Starchy Foods
   1½ cup chicken broth = a Freebie (Bouillon, a roughly
      comparable food, is on the Freebie list.)
   1 egg = ½ Meat/Poultry/Fish
   3 tbsp white wine = approx ½ A Bonus
   ⅔ cup cooked rice = 2 Breads/Cereals/Starchy Foods

3. Total the portions from each food group:

   3 Meat/Poultry/Fish + ½ Meat/Poultry/Fish = 3½
      Meat/Poultry/Fish portions;
   4½ A Bonus + ½ A Bonus = 5 A Bonus; and
   1 Breads/Cereals/Starchy Foods + 2 Breads/Cereals/
      Starchy Foods = 3 Breads/Cereals/Starchy Foods.

4. No portions need to be rounded.
5. Determine the number of Setpoint portions in each serving (this recipe serves three):

   3½ Meat/Poultry/Fish portions divided by 3 servings = 1⅙, or 1 Meat/Poultry/Fish portion
      (remember to round to the nearest half) per serving;
   5 A Bonus divided by 3 servings = 1⅔ A Bonus, or,
      rounding, 1½ A Bonus;

3 Breads/Cereals/Starchy Foods portions divided by
   3 servings = 1 Breads/Cereals/Starchy Foods portion per serving; and
1½ Vegetables portions divided by 3 servings = ½
   Vegetables portion per serving.
Setpoint portions for one serving of chicken vegetable
   casserole: 1 Meat/Poultry/Fish, 1½ A Bonus, 1
   Breads/Cereals/Starchy Foods, ½ Vegetables.

# Tips to Make Determining Portions Easier:

◊ Remember to include all fractional portions (2 tbsp
chopped onion = ¼ Vegetables portion). The
Measurement Conversion Table on p. 133 will
make it easy to calculate fractional portions.

◊ Refer to the Setpoint Guide to Ingredients on p.
132, which lists Setpoint portions for common
recipe ingredients.

◊ Pasta and rice absorb water during cooking, which
increases their volume; measure these foods *after*
cooking. As a quick guide, remember that 1 cup
dry regular rice = approximately 3 cups cooked;
1 cup dry instant rice = 2 cups cooked; 1 cup dry
spaghetti, fettuccine, linguini = 1½ cups cooked;
1 cup dry pasta, macaroni = 2½ cups cooked.

◊ Don't forget to make use of Freebies, such as
broth, bouillon, mustard, lemon juice, soy sauce,
herbs and spices. They can often replace high-
calorie flavorings. Experiment with them in cooking.

# Do's and Don'ts for Successful Portion Control

DO practice the dietary principles of balance, variety, and moderation when making your food choices—even among the Bonus Foods.

DO combine exercise with portion control to help you reach your desired weight goal.

DO drink plenty of fluids every day—water or low-calorie beverages. It will help fill you up; more important, it will replace fluids lost while exercising.

DO space your meals throughout the day instead of eating one big meal. Ideal is three small-to-moderate meals and one or more snacks.

DO carry a portion-control record with you each day and check off the food-group portions as you eat them. Writing down the specific foods you eat will help you include more variety in your daily menu.

DO eat all portions specified from the first five groups in order to meet daily nutritional requirements.

DO measure or weigh everything at first.

DON'T substitute between basic food groups.

DON'T go below 1200 calories without consulting your doctor.

DON'T eat the same foods all the time.

# Chapter Six

# Exercise

Now you are ready to begin the most important part of the Setpoint plan—the daily exercise that will lower your setpoint and allow you to keep weight off permanently.

I realize that some chronic dieters may not be convinced yet. Because the Setpoint Diet eating plan itself is so well-balanced and so easy to follow, you may be telling yourself, "I don't really need to exercise." If so, I'm afraid you are just fooling yourself. It is true that the eating plan by itself is extremely nutritious and so varied that you won't feel deprived, and you will probably even lose weight on it alone—for a while. If you don't lower your setpoint, however, you will not keep the weight off. And you will *not* lower your setpoint unless you exercise.

You may imagine that exercise is a sweaty, uncomfortable business, but that is probably because you have never felt the warm glow that comes after physical activity. You may perspire, yes, but this is a healthy sign indicating that your body is working the way it was meant to. Countless Setpointers have noted that they feel more energetic and healthy or, as one woman put it, "more normal," once they begin Setpoint exercise.

As you continue to exercise regularly, something else may happen—something you may not even imagine now. You may find that you come to *like* exercise and even look forward to it!

You may find, especially if you have been inactive for many years, a new sense of pride in yourself, in your body and what it is capable of doing.

So even if you've never so much as walked around the block in the past, I suggest that you give Setpoint exercising a try. No matter how out-of-shape you are, there are activities that are right for you and that will allow you to progress safely to higher levels of fitness.

You may want to consult a physician before beginning your exercise program; I strongly recommend it if you are more than 50 pounds overweight, are over 40, have been sedentary for many years, or have a history of heart disease or other medical condition that may make exercising inappropriate.

## Aerobic Exercise

You may have heard the term "aerobic" exercise and wondered what it means. Aerobic exercises are those moderate activities we have been talking about, the ones that will form the core of your Setpoint exercise program.

Aerobic exercising not only lowers your setpoint but also improves the fitness of your heart and blood vessels—your cardiovascular system.

The word aerobic literally means "with air." Aerobic exercise is sustained activity during which oxygen is continuously supplied to your muscles by your heart and lungs. Aerobic fitness is promoted by activities in which you use your large muscles (arms, legs, buttocks), in which your heart beats quickly, you breathe deeply, and you may perspire. In such exercises you are literally exercising your lungs and your heart (which is the most important muscle in your body). Among the most popular aerobic exercises are jogging, vigorous walking, swimming, aerobic dancing, and biking.

In order to lower your setpoint, you must perform aerobic activities *five times a week* (and lighter activities the other two days). This is important for both psychological and physiological reasons. Numerous studies have suggested that five is the optimum number of days each week to engage in aerobic exercise. Fewer than five, and the setpoint either will not be lowered or will be changed only minimally. More than five days of moderate aerobic exercise may be too much: certainly your body needs some time to rest and recover from stress. Psychologically, too, people appear to do better on a five-day-a-week regimen of aerobics, which allows some flexibility. Bear in mind that your setpoint will not be lowered faster if you exceed the recommended amount of exercise—but you could become exhausted or possibly even injured.

Remember: you should exercise every day. But on two days a week, choose a less strenuous exercise.

## Exercising at the Right Rate

The rate at which your heart should beat during exercise is determined in part by your age, but this does not mean that everyone of the same age should do the same exercises at the same intensity. Far from it. Your choice of exercise depends on a number of factors. One of the most important is your physical condition at the time you begin to exercise. Also important is your heredity—different people have different capacities for different activities. And of course your own likes and dislikes are crucial in picking activities that you will be able to stay with.

To get the full benefits of exercise, you need to exercise vigorously so your heart rate rises. Why? Consider an example: suppose you take 15 minutes to stroll to the bus stop two blocks away; you pause to look in store windows and talk to neighbors. When you arrive at the bus stop, your heart is beating at about its normal rate and you don't feel at all tired or out of breath. This means that while you may have moved your body two blocks, you have not *exercised*.

As you will see on page 61, there are numerous activities for you to choose from. For your five-day-a-week aerobic activities, choose from those that you can, with practice, perform for 30 continuous minutes at a level of

## Some Setpoint Exercises

Here are examples of Moderate (A) and Light (B) exercises that you can consider incorporating into your Setpoint plan. The activities should be performed continuously for 30 minutes. Some activities that are often performed strenuously enough to be on the A list (volleyball, tennis, dancing) are placed instead on the B list because they are usually performed on a stop-and-go basis.

| A | B |
| --- | --- |
| Running | Walking (2 mph) |
| Walking briskly (4 mph) | Performing light calisthenics |
| Bicycling | Playing tennis |
| Stationary bicycling | Playing golf |
| Running in place | Bowling |
| Aerobic dancing | Playing volleyball |
| Performing moderate calisthenics | Playing touch football |
| Skipping rope | Ice skating—leisure |
| Swimming | Roller skating—leisure |
| Rowing | Hiking |
| Playing handball | Dancing |
| Playing basketball—full court | Doing housework |
| Skiing, cross-country | Mowing the lawn |
| Canoeing | Raking leaves |
| Lifting weights | Waxing floors |
| Practicing martial arts | Gardening |
|  | Performing yoga |

effort that increases your heart rate to its "target zone."

In the target zone, your heart beats faster than when it's at rest. It's not beating so fast that you are aware of a thumping in your side or are completely out of breath, nor is it beating so slowly that you can keep it up "forever." As a general rule of thumb, you should do your five-days-a-week aerobic exercise at a level of effort at which you can easily carry on a conversation (if you have no one to talk to, try singing) but at which you clearly feel that you are expending effort. If you are too out-of-breath to talk, you are exercising too strenuously. If you feel no effect at all, however, your exercising is not strenuous enough.

Those are pretty general descriptions—you'll need to compute your heart-rate target zone more precisely if you want to get the most from your Setpoint exercise program. In addition, learning to compute your target zone and monitor your heart rate can help you guard against exercising too vigorously.

# How to Find Your Heart-Rate Target Zone

You can compute your own personal target zone's upper and lower limits using the simple formula in the box on page 63. You should aim to maintain your heart rate within those limits throughout your half-hour aerobic exercise periods. If your heart rate goes above the target range, you are exercising too strenuously; if it goes below the target zone, pick up the pace a little.

You'll also need to know how to monitor your heart rate. There are several ways to do this—most people I know think it's easiest to do by feeling the pulse in the carotid artery on either side of the neck. This major artery carries blood to the head and can be located by sliding the tips of your extended fingers to the side of your Adam's apple.

To determine if you are exercising within your target zone, stop doing your exercise periodically—every 2 to 4 minutes—and take your pulse. Because the heart rate drops quickly after you stop exercising (the more fit you are the more quickly it drops), it is best to count the pulse beats for only 10 seconds and then immediately resume exercising. Multiply your 10-second count by six: this is the heart rate per minute at which you are exercising. If it is above or below your target zone, adjust your efforts accordingly. After a few weeks, you will probably be able to "feel" whether you are in the target range.

---

### Determining Your Target Heart-Rate Zone

*A Four-Step Formula*

1. Subtract your age from 220.
2. From the result, subtract your resting heart rate— the rate that your heart beats per minute after you have been inactive for a while.
3. Multiply the result of step 2 by .5 and .7.
4. Add your resting heart rate to each result of step 3.

This will give you the high and low of the heart-rate zone at which you should aim when exercising.

*Example*

For a 40-year-old individual whose resting heart rate is 76.

1. $220-40 = 180$
2. $180-76 = 104$
3. $104 \times .5 = 52$
   $104 \times .7 = 72.8$
4. $52 + 76 = 128$
   $72.8 + 76 = 148.8$

Thus, this person's target heart-rate zone is 128 to 149 beats per minute.

---

# Choosing Activities That Are Right for You

Dr. George Sheehan, a cardiologist who is sometimes called the guru of runners, does not, surprisingly, recommend his favorite activity for everyone. Rather, he emphasizes that each of us is different, with different needs and likes.

Take another look at the chart on page 61. It lists two levels of exercise—A (moderate) and B (light)—that you can choose from. Look the lists over—identify those activities that you enjoy or that you have perhaps always wanted to try. Dr. Sheehan recommends that you think of exercise as a time to be playful. If you are a confirmed nonexerciser, think back to the last time in your life that you *were* active. Did you like to ride your bicycle when you were a child? If so, then stationary or mobile bicycling might form the core of your exercise program. What about skating? Swimming?

Choose your five-times-a-week aerobic exercise from activities such as those found on the A list. You can choose to do the same activity (e.g. swimming) five times a week, or you can alternate. For example: Monday, Wednesday, and Saturday, brisk walking; Tuesday and Thursday, swimming. For the remaining two days, choose from the lighter kind of activities included on the B list.

If you are extremely overweight or have not exercised in a very long time, it is best to begin with walking. This is because you can easily control the rate at which you walk, so you don't tax your present degree of conditioning. As you get into shape, you can increase your level of activity.

## A Activities

Engage in these types of activities for 30 consecutive minutes five times per week. Make sure your heart rate gets into the target zone and stays there. Before you start, however, warm up with some stretching; don't forget to cool down, too, when you're finished. Let's take a look at some of the A activities:

Walking  You might consider starting with—and even staying with—this excellent form of exercise, particularly if you have been sedentary for a long time or are very overweight (more than 25 percent over ideal weight). As I have emphasized before, just strolling down the street will not suffice to lower your setpoint. Instead, you must walk for 30 consecutive minutes at a pace that elevates your heart rate into your target zone.

Choose a route that has a minimum number of intersections or walk in a park. If you live near a school or municipal track, do your walking on the track. Many joggers and walkers use them.

Wear a pair of good running shoes. Street shoes (especially those with high heels) do *not* give your feet the proper protection and support for recreational walking. Your entire exercise program probably depends upon your feet—so look after them!

Jogging/Running This is a good exercise for most people. It quickly raises your heart rate and it's easy. You can jog anywhere, and jogging can easily be phased into a walking program as you become more fit.

As with walking, if you decide to make jogging part of your program, I strongly urge you to invest in a pair of good running shoes. There are many types available now, in all sizes, for both men and women, and some are quite attractive. Apart from shoes there is no investment required, though you might want to get brightly colored sweat pants or even a stylish warm-up suit. Wearing the right gear can get you in the mood and make you feel like a track star, even if you're a plodder! If you expect to walk or jog along a road, be sure to wear reflecting tape or other devices to make you more visible to motorists.

Swimming This is another excellent exercise which strengthens the upper body and provides a good aerobic workout. It is less stressful on the joints than jogging can sometimes be. If you live near a swimming club or belong to a gym that has a pool, swimming might well be a good exercise to include in your program.

Cycling This is an activity that can be enjoyed by people of all ages. It is less stressful on the joints than running, although people with knee problems may find cycling uncomfortable. It is important to get a good bike that's the right size for you. A three-speed bike should be all you need, unless you plan to be doing a lot of biking on hills. Depending on where you live, cycling can be combined as exercise and transportation.

Stationary Cycling   This is one of the most practical of exercises, because it can be performed in the privacy of your home, at any time and regardless of weather conditions. The only drawbacks are that a good bike is rather expensive and that you must have room to set it up. Many Setpointers I have talked to like to keep the bike in the same room with the TV so they can exercise while watching their favorite programs. Others read.

Aerobic Dance   This has become one of the most popular exercises for both men and women. Classes are offered at many Y's and gyms throughout the country. If you truly hate to exercise, aerobic dance may be for you! Once you have learned the routines, you can enjoy performing them at home to your favorite records.

## A Note on Outdoor Exercise.

Any activity that you perform outdoors during the day—walking, jogging, tennis, swimming, cycling—exposes you to the rays of the sun. Many experts now believe that premature wrinkling and spotting and other degenerative changes that can lead to skin cancer may be caused in part by exposure to the sun. If you are concerned about such changes or want to prevent sunburn, it is a good idea to apply a protective sunscreen to all exposed parts of your body. The safest products for all skin types are those that are labeled SPF (Sun Protection Factor) 15 or higher.

## B Activities

You should engage in B type activities two days each week (and feel free to vary your choices from week to week). As you can see from the chart on page 61, a wide range of recreational and leisure activities are included. By themselves, the B exercises will not be sufficient to lower your setpoint, either because they are not strenuous enough to get your heart into the target zone (golf, raking leaves) or because they are stop-and-go activities that probably won't keep your heart in the target zone for 30 consecutive minutes (tennis, volleyball).

## Getting Started

How you start obviously depends on your degree of conditioning. If you're an inactive person, a two-block sprint for the bus may leave you panting from exhaustion, scarcely able to talk, your heart pounding so heavily that you can hear it in your ears. A person who is more fit, however, might have no problem running those two blocks. She might arrive ahead of you, breathing nearly as slowly as if she were just strolling. This is because her heart is now trained and can efficiently pump blood under conditions of sudden stress.

The following section discusses some points you should keep in mind when you're planning to start a Setpoint exercise program—whether you're a beginning, intermediate, or advanced exerciser.

Beginner  You qualify as a beginner if you have been inactive in recent years or you are very overweight (more than 25 percent over ideal weight).

If you are a beginner, you need to start slowly and gradually increase your fitness. This is especially important for people over 40. It should take most people about six to eight weeks to get into shape. If it takes you less time or more time, don't worry; work at your own pace.

Weeks 1 and 2  Begin by performing your A activities in several 5-minute periods, resting the same amount of time in between. (Thus, if your activity is walking, walk briskly for five minutes, rest or walk more slowly for five minutes, then walk again, rest again.) Don't worry that you are not performing a total of 30 minutes yet—you are still conditioning yourself! Be sure to take your pulse often to see that you are in the target zone. If you feel no challenge at all, pick up the pace or increase the length of each exercise period. If you find yourself out of breath or experience pain in the midchest, slow down. (Recurring chest pain warrants the attention of a physician.)

**Weeks 3 and 4** Increase your exercise periods to 7 minutes each. Pay close attention to your breathing and heart rate; adjust the intensity of your activity as appropriate.

**Weeks 5 and 6** Increase your exercise periods to 10 minutes. Monitor as before.

**Weeks 7 and 8** Increase the amount of time you perform the activity until you are approaching 30 nonstop minutes.

The above schedule is a guide only. Use your heart rate and the way you feel to help you decide when to increase the intensity of your exercises. Don't try to do too much too soon—that will result in fatigue and even possible injury.

**Intermediate** Begin at this level if you are somewhat active (perhaps a "weekend athlete") or you are not severely overweight.

Follow the guidelines for beginners but start with the regimen suggested for weeks 3 and 4. You should be able to reach nonstop activity around the sixth week.

**Advanced** Start at this level if you already have been exercising at least three days a week.

Perform your activity nonstop for 30 consecutive minutes. But don't overdo it. For example, if jogging is a part of your program, you might want to slow to a walk occasionally for the first week or two until you have built up your stamina. Again, let your body be your guide.

At least initially, stop every 10 minutes or so to monitor your pulse rate. If it is too fast, slow down or walk for a few minutes; if it is too slow, increase your effort.

## Four Easy Steps

To summarize, here are the four simple steps you follow to begin your own individualized exercise program.

Step One   Determine your target heart-rate zone. (See page 63.)

Step Two   Decide which exercise(s) from group A you will perform five times a week. To prevent boredom, be sure to make your program flexible—vary and combine your activities! (See page 61.)

Step Three   Choose one or more activities from group B to be performed twice a week. (See page 61.)

Step Four   Decide on your present conditioning level—beginning, intermediate, or advanced—and then get started!

## When to Exercise

This is as individual a matter as choosing which exercises are right for you. Some people prefer to exercise in the morning "because it gives me energy for the whole day," as one woman I know says. Others like to exercise in the morning just to "get it over with!"

In the corporate exercise program at General Foods, groups of employees get together during their lunch period for a brisk 30-minute walk. "It wakes me up," reports a secretary. "I really find it invigorating."

If you prefer to exercise at night and if your program includes jogging, walking, or bicycling, be sure to take safety precautions. Wear a reflective vest and shoe strips. Run against the direction of traffic; but bicycle *with* the traffic.

You can perform your B activities at any time—even right after a meal—but it is best not to do A activities until an hour or two after eating. This is because a great deal of your blood supply is devoted to digestion after a meal. If you suddenly begin to work out and divert that blood to your skeletal muscles, painful stomach cramps could result.

Some Setpointers report that moderate exercise *before* a meal makes them less hungry; you may observe that, too. Experiment to see what exercise schedule is best for you.

# What about Bad Weather?

One reason I urge you to adopt a variety of activities for your program is so inclement weather won't serve as a barrier (or an excuse!) to keep you from exercising.

You might want to consider investing in a good piece of aerobic exercise equipment for use indoors: a stationary cycle, a trampoline, a cross-country simulator, even a rowing machine. You might have to spend a few hundred dollars—a cheap piece of equipment is no bargain. Or look for a good piece of used equipment.

Of course, you can walk or jog in any kind of weather short of a heavy blizzard, and many Setpointers do just that. In fact, there are several excellent weatherproof warm-up suits that will protect you from rain and snow and keep you warm.

# Exercise for a Lifetime

After you have been on your exercise program for a few weeks, you will notice amazing improvements in how you look and feel. If you are like most Setpointers, you will find that you look forward to exercise as one of the high points of your day. But even if you are like John McGuckin, who maintains that he enjoys jogging only "when I'm finished," you will probably be so pleased with the results that you won't consider giving it up.

Remember that the social side of exercise can be important to the success of your program. Some Setpointers exercise with their spouses—or even with their entire families! Try to find buddies to run or swim with. And by all means let each of your B activities be something that you particularly enjoy, not something you do just because it is good for you. If you have always wanted to learn a sport—badminton, say—now is the time. Joining an exercise group or a sports club can help you get into new activities.

Remember that you are not only losing weight; you

are also improving the fitness of your body and mind, approaching the healthy ideal nature intended for you.

## Exercise Do's and Don'ts

DO drink plenty of water to replace that lost during exercise.

DO exercise in your target heart zone.

DO exercise seven days a week, but perform A activities no more than five times per week.

DO exercise for 30 consecutive minutes.

DO buy good running shoes if your A exercises include walking or jogging.

DO consider consulting a physician before beginning your exercise program, certainly if you are more than 25 percent overweight, are past forty, have been sedentary in recent years, or have a medical condition that may make exercise inappropriate.

DO warm up before exercising and cool down after exercising.

DON'T overdo any exercise.

DON'T let occasional "off" days discourage you—your body is still getting used to its new activity level.

DON'T do A exercises just after a meal (wait at least an hour or two).

DON'T exercise if you are running a fever or feel so sick that you can't go to work.

Chapter Seven

# Adopting Setpoint Smoothly

The hardest part of any new regimen is always the first few days or weeks. This is true for at least two reasons. First, it's easy to get discouraged because the payoff—a new, slimmer you—seems to lie so far in the future. Second, learning anything new requires effort and commitment. You are getting used to portion control; you are getting used to working daily exercise into your life.

After a few days or weeks, however, it will become much easier to stay with the routine. You are losing weight! You are feeling good about yourself! What has happened? The Setpoint Diet has become a part of your life; practicing portion control and exercising have become automatic—as natural as brushing your teeth.

Until you reach that point, you may need some help to keep going. In this chapter we will take a look at a number of devices and strategies that have been used by other successful Setpointers to keep themselves on track even on those occasional off days.

# Why People Sometimes Drop Out

Although the Setpoint Diet has helped a great many people to lose weight, some inevitably drop out. This usually occurs for predictable reasons.

First, some people drop out because they feel the diet isn't working for them. They feel they are not losing weight fast enough. Almost always it turns out that they have not been exercising faithfully or are not using portion control properly.

In other cases, dropouts have occurred for the opposite reason: the dieter has become so zealous that he or she is getting too few calories or is overdoing the exercise to the point of exhaustion.

To be sure this does not happen to you, remember the cornerstones of the program: balance, variety, and moderation. Bear in mind, too, that you did not gain all that weight overnight—it will take you some time to lose it safely. The heavier you now are, the longer it will take. Remember also the diet alone will not lower your setpoint: only regular, moderate exercise will both lower your setpoint and diminish your appetite.

Another reason sometimes given for dropping out of the program or not following it exactly is that portion control is "too complicated." I'm sorry, but I cannot buy that as an excuse! It is true that it takes some planning, especially at first, and perhaps a little extra time in the kitchen while you are learning the portions. As Angela Doering puts it, "It's like learning how to drive. After four or five weeks I had it down pat. Now it's automatic." The Setpoint Diet promises you a lifetime of healthy eating and a slimmer body in return for a very small commitment on your part.

One of the most often heard excuses for straying from the diet is interruptions by vacation or business travel. It is true that travel can upset your routine; also, when you are far from home it is sometimes difficult to continue with an exercise or diet regimen. However, if you are honest with yourself you will recognize that travel is no excuse. The Setpoint Diet is so generous and allows so many different foods that eating in restaurants does not need to be a problem (for tips on eating in restaurants, see chapter 12). And as for exercising—what better time than when you are on vacation, presumably relaxed and perhaps in a resort area where exercise is encouraged? And on business trips you can plan to stay in hotels having exercise facilities.

I would caution you against *beginning* the Setpoint Diet while on vacation, because it would be easier to begin in familiar surroundings. But while you're away there is no reason not to continue a program you've already started. For tips on how to continue Setpoint when traveling or on vacation, see chapter 12.

Still another common excuse is that there "simply isn't enough time" to work a half-hour's worth of exercise into the daily routine. Let's face it: thirty minutes is only a fraction of your day, and the benefits you receive are so substantial—lost weight, increased energy, improved self-esteem—that the amount of time you put in seems a small investment indeed. Besides, you can always make time for anything you really want to do. And often you can combine your exercise with other daily activities. Debra Kaiser, for example, a busy scientist whose husband joined her on the diet, found an ingenious way to prepare Setpoint meals and get her exercise at the same time: "Once when I was really busy I took my exercise bike in the kitchen and set it up by the stove," she says. "When Mike got home at first he thought I was crazy. Then he decided I was *really* devoted to Setpoint!"

Of course you needn't go as far as Debra did, but the point is that if you are serious about losing weight on Setpoint, you *can* find a way.

## Suggestions for Success

Enlist Your Family   The reason you have decided to go on the Setpoint Diet is that you care about your health and appearance. This is important to keep in mind: you are doing something very special for yourself, and you have every right to feel good about it! The more support you can create for yourself in your environment, the easier it will be to continue toward your goals.

The first, most obvious place to look for support is your family. A research study showed that male coronary patients on exercise programs who had the support of their wives did far better than those without such support. Similar results have been reported by many couples who have followed Setpoint together. One woman, for example, wrote me that she had been planning to drop out, but "my husband encouraged me to continue."

Inform family members that you are going on the Setpoint Diet. Explain what it is and how it works. Describing the diet and its principles can benefit you, too—explaining it to someone else is one of the best ways of learning it thoroughly.

Don't be afraid to ask for the support of loved ones. Since the Setpoint Diet includes all foods that you might conceivably wish to eat, you won't have to ask a spouse or child to keep forbidden foods out of your sight, although you might want to ask them to be considerate about snacking in your presence. It can help tremendously if your spouse or one of your children can join you in your half-hour exercise program—many successful Setpointers have made daily exercise a family routine. This can be a time for togetherness.

Get a Buddy   Another possibility is to get a buddy. Whenever one of you is feeling down, the other can be encouraging. As often as possible, plan and eat your meals together; try to exercise together. If your activity is biking or walking, you will be amazed at how quickly the time passes when you do it together, talking as you go.

Form a Group   One reason for the success of such diet groups as Weight Watchers and TOPS is that most people find it easier to engage in new behavior in a group setting. These and other groups have a good record of initial weight loss; however, once participants drop out they tend to regain weight unless they continue to engage in daily exercise.

Following the Setpoint Diet also can be easier with group support. If you find it difficult to stick with the diet at the beginning, I urge you to try to form a group. Where can you find one? Perhaps in your own neighborhood; put up a notice on the bulletin board in the supermarket. Or see if you can form a Setpoint group at work. Comparing weekly weight loss is also beneficial—more than one Setpointer has remarked that it's "easier to stick to it if someone else will know your weight."

One successful neighborhood group was formed, almost by accident, by my wife's cousin. She began her program by walking every evening, usually with her husband or daughter. At first, she told me, her friends and neighbors thought she was wasting her time. Gradually, though, they began to notice her weight loss, and one by one they began to join her. Now, in what I think of as the Pied Piper syndrome, she has become the leader of a group of seven or eight dedicated Setpointers, all of whom meet for an evening walk through their Pennsylvania town.

Keep Records   This is important, especially in the early stages of the diet. Until you are completely familiar with Setpoint details, it is a good idea to make several copies of the Portion Control Record (see pages 48–52) and carry one with you each day. These charts have spaces to record your food intake for the day; enter the specific food you eat for each food group portion. This is a handy way of making sure you get enough variety. Make sure to use the chart that's appropriate to your calorie level.

Some successful dieters also like to keep a graph charting weekly progress in weight loss. A sample graph on p.77 shows how the subject progresses in her goal to lose 20 pounds. On those days when you are feeling discouraged, this visible record of your progress can be just the stimulus you need to keep going.

Another way to chart your progress is to record key measurements at the beginning of the program. Measure your chest, waist, thighs, hips, upper arms—and keep track of changes on a weekly basis. Since the combined exercise-diet program builds lean tissue at the expense of fat, you may see dramatic changes in these measurements before weight loss shows up on the scale.

## Charting Weekly Progress

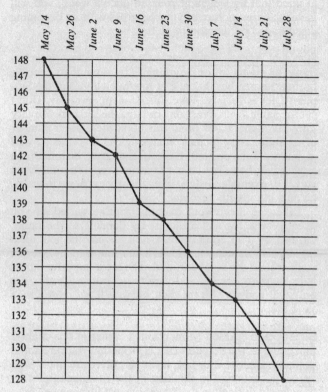

A 20-pound loss is recorded on this homemade chart. Such visual records are important morale-boosters for many dieters.

<u>Don't Get Addicted to the Scale</u>   There is no reason to weigh yourself more than once a week. Of course, this a very individual matter, but many dieters make something of a fetish of weighing themselves each morning or evening (or both!). The trouble with this is that the weight display can often be misleading: a particularly heavy or salty meal the night before can cause water retention that may panic you into thinking that you are failing.

It is perfectly all right to weigh yourself daily, but bear in mind that by weighing yourself once a week, you will have a clearer picture of your progress without becoming discouraged by temporary shifts.

<u>Don't Let Yourself Get Bored</u>   One of the surest prescriptions for giving up on anything is to allow it to become boring. Remember that one of the touchstones of the Setpoint Diet is variety. Take this concept seriously. Don't eat the same foods every day or have the same meal every Tuesday night. Later on in this book there are a number of exciting, tasty recipes, featuring old favorites as well as international cuisine. Experiment. Try a dish that you have never had. Try an old favorite prepared a different way. For example, instead of eggplant or veal parmigiana, try making it with zucchini.

Likewise, keep your exercise routine varied. If you usually walk for half an hour, try dancing to the radio. Or walk by a different route. Learn to combine activities: try aerobic dancing for 15 minutes followed by a brisk walk around the neighborhood. The most important thing is to keep excitement and variety in your program—not only will you stay on the diet, but you'll put more fun in your life.

<u>Be Good to Yourself</u>   I mentioned earlier in this chapter that going on the Setpoint Diet is proof that you care about yourself. Believe it or not, however, there are many who are so accustomed to thinking of their families first that they find it difficult to do something just for themselves—like becoming a Setpointer. Nobody has put this feeling better than Mary Grimm. At 42, the mother of two teenagers, with a working spouse and a new career, Mary is beginning to learn that she must take care of herself, too, especially when she is under stress. She has recently joined a health fitness center, "in order to impose a routine in my life," she says. "I have also told my supervisor that I am under stress. I know now that I, as many overweight people, have to learn not to please others to the point that it exhausts my reserves of energy. I plan to spend time on pleasing myself and taking care of myself."

This is good advice for anyone. Exercise is, after all, something you do just for yourself. Give yourself some special time each day. You deserve it! And be proud of what you have accomplished.

<u>Reward Yourself</u>  Establish short-term goals and plan to reward yourself when you meet them. For example, give yourself a special treat each time you lose 5 pounds—buy yourself something: a scarf, a book, a record. No matter how much weight you want to lose, you have to do it in increments. Giving yourself a pat on the back each time you achieve a step toward your goal can boost your self-esteem and strengthen your resolve. Reward yourself for success in exercising, too. For example, you might decide to walk one mile five times a week for four weeks; when you have done that, buy yourself a present.

## Sticking with the Setpoint Diet

<u>Plan</u>  If I had to give one key to success in following portion control, it is to plan ahead. Nearly all the successful Setpointers have mentioned that they do this, although all note that it becomes much less a conscious process after a while.

Angela Doering, a secretary, plans lunch and dinner each morning with her husband, who has lost 21 pounds on Setpoint. "We try to think about variety," she says. "It's never anything elaborate, but it seems that just discussing it forces us to think about what we'll eat during the day. It keeps us both from avoiding instant gratification or last-minute snacks."

Tony Arcuri, a 63-year-old electrician, also plans meals with his wife each day. "The main thing we plan for is sweets," he says. "We both like being able to have our favorite 'weakness' on the diet, and we prefer to have it in the evening. It helps that we plan together. I know that if I have cookies at lunch I'll have to watch her have hers at dinner—and that's no fun!"

Eat Frequently   Snacking can be an integral part of the
Setpoint Diet. Plan your snacks; they make it easier to
get from meal to meal. The tastier and better-looking your
snacks are, the better. You might prepare celery sticks
stuffed with herbed low-fat cottage cheese or slice a small
apple (1 Fruits portion) and arrange it on a plate alter-
nating with thin slices of swiss cheese (1 oz = 1 Milk/
Dairy products). If you feel that you must have some
"bulk," make some popcorn (3 cups popped = 1 Breads/
Cereals/Starchy Foods)—sprinkle it with rosemary for a
different and delicious treat!

Make each snack an "event" and you won't get hungry
or bored.


Be Patient with Yourself   For many Setpointers, exercise
seems more difficult than dieting. This is not because it
really is any harder, and it's not because—as some people
allege—it takes so much time. The real reason is that
many people find exercising unfamiliar and perhaps a little
daunting.

Don't expect miracles from yourself! If you haven't
exercised in many years, you will not be ready to run a
marathon within a few short weeks. Whatever your activity, do it briskly enough to raise your heart rate but not
so strenuously that you are left panting and exhausted.
As you will see, the results of exercise do become appar-
ent very quickly; within a very few days you will notice
your stamina increasing and you may even see a decrease
in your waistline—even before a change shows up on the
scales.

Try not to be self-conscious. If you have been overweight for some time, you may imagine that other people
will laugh when they find out what you are doing. Don't
let yourself feel that way. Chances are no one is even
noticing you. And if they are, they are probably thinking
something like "Good for her (or him)!"

If you are too embarrassed to exercise in public, you
might try what I call Setpoint by Moonlight—do your
exercise after dark. Or take up an exercise that you can
perform privately, like stationary bicycling.

Compete with Yourself   This technique is a variation on setting goals, and while it won't work for everyone, it can be effective if you are competitive by nature. Michael Coyne, who lost 28 pounds on Setpoint in only 12 weeks, chose jogging as his exercise. "What kept me going was trying to surpass myself," he reports. "Like, first it was a big deal to run half a mile, then one mile, then two. Now I'm pretty fit and I set time goals. I push myself to see if I can run the same distance a little faster each time. It's a way of keeping going."

You needn't jog to compete with yourself. If you are riding a stationary bike, you can aim at a certain number of miles. Or try to walk a favorite neighborhood route faster than you did last night.

Exercise to Music   Dancing is not the only Setpoint activity that involves music. You can do many other types of exercise—jumping rope, jogging, stationary cycling—to records, tapes, or the radio. One young woman made a 30-minute tape of some of her favorite songs. She jogs until the tape has run out, and she reports that the time speeds by.

Dress Up   The increased popularity of exercising has resulted in a wider selection of attractive exercise clothes. They are available in all colors of the rainbow, and you don't have to spend a lot of money. Make an occasion of your exercise—buy some nice T-shirts and colorful sweat pants. Invest in a good pair of running shoes (especially if your activity is walking or jogging).

Not only will such gear make you look and feel good (and serious), but spending the money may give you an added incentive to continue the program.

Distract Yourself   If you feel that exercising is truly boring, then find a way to distract yourself. Exercise while you are doing something else. As I mentioned before, music can help. You can also watch TV (particularly easy when using a stationary exercise bicycle, as is reading). For other exercises, use your portable radio to listen to the news or an interesting public affairs program. Put on language tapes and work toward your goal of reading Camus in French. Or use the time to plan your menu, memorize poetry, or rehearse a speech you plan to deliver.

Boredom can be your worst enemy. Think positively and concentrate on the benefits—and you should seldom find exercise tedious.

Fool Yourself   On those days when you just don't feel up to it or you think you just don't have enough time to exercise—fool yourself! Begin to exercise, telling yourself, "I'll just do this for five minutes. If I'm still feeling bad (or worried about time) I'll stop."

Usually, you will find that just getting started was half the battle and finishing is easier than you had imagined.

Join a Gym   Finally, you might join a gym or exercise class. Not only can the financial commitment provide an incentive to keep going, but you will benefit from the support of others who are at the same level of conditioning as you are. Furthermore, you won't have an excuse to skip exercise when it is cold or raining. Many Y's and health clubs offer classes in aerobic and other exercise at all levels.

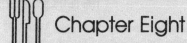 Chapter Eight

# A Treasury of Tips for Successful Setpointing

## Changing Your Attitude toward Food

Many dieters employ behavior-modification techniques aimed at changing their attitudes and behavior toward food. Countless studies show that behavior modification works.

Although group support is often involved in behavior modification, you can practice many of the techniques alone. Behavior modification usually focuses on one or more of the following three steps: self-monitoring, stimulus control, and learning how to modify actual behavior. Through self-monitoring, you recognize the circumstances under which you are likely to overeat; then you alter or regulate these circumstances to facilitate a change in behavior. For example, a man who just can't pass up fast foods might realize that he tends to overeat when standing at a food counter. He might train himself to eat only while sitting. It is much less threatening for him to concede, "Okay, I can never again eat standing up—but I can still have ice cream."

You can employ this technique yourself. Keep a notebook or simply make mental notes of situations that are most tempting for you and then take steps to modify them.

Suppose your favorite snack is potato chips, but you find it impossible to stop eating them before finishing a whole bag. One solution is to give up chips forever. A more realistic way of dealing with the problem might be to ask your spouse or a friend to open the chips for you and put them in small baggies of a few chips each, which you can then eat for a snack. (15 chips = 1 B Bonus.)

Perhaps without realizing it, you have probably used some behavior-modification techniques in the past. Keeping a food diary is a form of self-monitoring, designed to heighten your awareness of your eating habits. Below are some other techniques that may help you to change your eating behavior for the better.

◊ Learn to eat slowly. Studies show that overweight people tend to eat quickly, gobbling up their food and scarcely tasting it. Try putting down your fork after every bite and chewing the food thoroughly, noting how it tastes. You may be surprised by subtleties in flavor you hadn't noticed before. Bear in mind that it takes about 20 minutes for your brain to get the message that you are full—and you don't want to overeat before that message is delivered!

◊ While you're still learning portion control, serve your meals on salad plates instead of dinner plates. That way, the food will fill the plate and you won't feel deprived.

◊ While you're at it, use your good china and silverware. Light candles and put on some soft music. Make each meal a special occasion, tranquil and appealing to all your senses. This will help keep you from feeling as if you are "on a diet."

◊ Take up a project such as needlework or model-building to keep your hands busy so you won't be tempted to munch when you get bored.

◊ Always eat at the table, and don't watch TV or read while you are eating. This way you concentrate only on the meal and enjoy it more. If you are doing something else while eating, you can easily lose track of how much food you have had.

◊ Use the kitchen only to prepare and eat meals. If you use it for something else—say, to write letters— you may be tempted to snack every time you go in.

◊ Plan and shop ahead. In the beginning it might even be helpful to buy on the weekend for the week ahead. You will thus avoid having to make hasty food decisions when you are in a rush.

◊ Don't cook more than you need at any one time so there won't be leftovers to tempt you (unless the leftovers are to be used for another meal).

# Tips for Planning and Preparing Meals

◊ Ask your spouse or children to put away groceries and/or clear the table if you can't resist snacking.

◊ Remove the skin and visible fat from chicken and visible fat from chops and steaks before cooking.

◊ Look for starchy vegetables such as peas, corn, and beans in the Breads/Cereals/Starchy Foods group.

◊ Use whipped butter or margarine or cream cheese; you can have half again as much by volume of the whipped variety as the regular kind.

◊ Cook bacon by placing it on a rack in a pan and bake it till it's crisp. The fat will end up in the pan, not in the bacon. Or cook it in the microwave on paper towels, which will absorb the fat.

◊ Always weigh meat, fish, and poultry *after* cooking. Four ounces of lean raw meat equals 3 ounces cooked.

◊ Have a good source of protein for breakfast: milk, eggs, meat, or cheese.

◊ Flavor vegetables and rice with lemon juice or rind or add herbs and spices—not butter.

◊ Use fresh fruit or fruit that is canned or frozen without sugar.

◊ Stretch mayonnaise or salad dressing by combining it with the low-calorie variety, or add lemon juice or yogurt.

◊ Roast, broil, or bake (and trim all visible fat) to cut down on extra calories. Scramble eggs in a no-stick pan.

◊ A tasty lower-calorie dip for vegetables can be made by adding herbs to low-fat cottage cheese, ricotta, or low-fat yogurt.

◊ If you like sandwiches but don't want to use two Breads/Cereals/Starchy Foods portions at one meal, try an open-faced sandwich or a pita pocket sandwich.

◊ When preparing soup, stews, or meat sauces, allow time to refrigerate so that fat will congeal and you can discard it.

◊ Buy tuna in water, not oil. It's lower in calories, but it costs (and tastes) the same.

◊ Although cornstarch has no more calories than flour, it has twice the thickening power.

◊ Buy a small food scale to weigh meats, fish, and cheese until you can recognize portion size at a glance.

◊ Likewise, use measuring spoons at first to teach yourself what two teaspoons of butter or mayonnaise look like when spread on bread. Do the same with salad dressing before you pour it on your salad.

◊ Using a measuring cup, pour 4 fluid ounces, 5 fluid ounces, and 8 fluid ounces of water into your favorite glasses at home. Take note of how each amount looks so you won't have to measure each time you have a beverage.

◊ When baking, experiment with cutting down on sugar and shortening in the recipe. In some recipes you can cut them by half—and not affect the flavor.

◊ When cooking oriental meals, cut down on rice and double up on vegetables. Use less oil in stir-frying.

◊ Don't add oil for browning or sautéing if something in the ingredients is fatty in itself.

◊ Put fresh herbs with low-fat cottage cheese or low-fat yogurt on baked potato, instead of sour cream or butter.

◊ Oregano makes a perfect no-calorie topping for tomatoes, while nutmeg is delicious grated over cooked spinach.

◊ Prepare deviled eggs with dry mustard and milk rather than mayonnaise.

◊ Instead of gravy, try cooking mushrooms in bouillon to serve over meat.

## Eating Tips

◊ Put a sauce or gravy on the side, then dip your food into it as you dine. You will eat much less of it this way.

◊ When eating out, ask for a small portion of dessert or share it with a companion.

◊ At breakfast, use low-fat milk instead of cream on cereal or in coffee. Remember that muffins and toast are in the Breads/Cereals/Starchy Foods group, while doughnuts and Danish are B Bonus foods.

◊ Snack on crunchy vegetables—zucchini, carrots, cucumbers, green beans.

◊ If you like fish, buy or order those that are lower in fat: cod, flounder, haddock, halibut, and sole; you're allowed four ounces instead of two ounces per portion.

◊ Beware of cocktails before dinner. All alcohol, including beer and wine, is on either the A or B Bonus lists. Club soda, seltzer, and mineral water are Freebies.

◊ When ordering chicken or turkey, you're allowed one extra ounce per portion if you request white meat instead of dark meat. Remember, eating the skin adds extra calories.

◊ Crave a crunch? Crushed ice with a diet drink (or fruit juice) poured over it looks pretty in a mug or cup. Eat it with a spoon.

## Exercise Tips

◊ If possible, schedule your light activity for after a meal.

◊ On the other hand, if you perform aerobic exercise just before your main meal of the day, you will have less appetite and be less tempted to overeat.

◊ Schedule your exercise period as if it were a business appointment. Don't let anything interfere with it.

◊ Whenever possible, incorporate exercise into your regular activities.

◊ To make your A exercise more enjoyable and stress-free, do gentle stretching exercises for 5 to 10 minutes before and after.

Refer back to chapters 6 and 7 for more exercise tips.

## Troubleshooting

Because the Setpoint Diet is so well balanced and so easy to follow, you should have few problems with it. However, here are some troubleshooting ideas—just in case.

## Following Portion Control and Exercising but Not Losing Weight

This does happen from time to time, particularly to people who were already exercising when they started the diet and to those who had only a very few pounds to lose.

If you find yourself in this situation, the first thing to do is to try the next-lower calorie level—but never go below 1200 calories without consulting your doctor.

Second, review your exercise program. Perhaps it is not challenging enough for you, and you need to increase the intensity (see chapter 6 for information on determining your exercise needs). Make sure that whatever your exercise plan, you are performing it continuously for 30 minutes a day.

## Losing Too Much Weight Too Rapidly

Although it can be a heady experience to lose weight rapidly, losing too rapidly—anything over, say, 3 or 4 pounds a week—is too much. Not only does it indicate water or muscle loss; it can leave you feeling weak.

If you find that you are losing too rapidly, try the next-higher calorie level of the diet. Check your exercise level, too. You may be performing more exercise than your body is accustomed to, which can result in exhaustion, depression, and injury. Moderate, not heavy, exercise is the key.

## Lost Weight but Suddenly Stopped; Hit a Plateau

The cause is often simple carelessness in following the Setpoint plan. Review your current food intake. Are you scrupulous about measuring portions? Are you eating the correct number of portions for your calorie level?

Perhaps you are failing to lose because you are getting insufficient exercise to affect your setpoint. Are you exercising for 30 consecutive minutes—every day? Remember that fewer than 30 minutes is not enough; although inadequate exercise will burn off calories, it will *not* lower your setpoint.

If you are certain that you are following both the portion control and the exercise programs correctly, then try dropping to the next-lower calorie level (but, again, don't go below 1200 calories without your doctor's supervision). Or increase the intensity of your exercise (see chapter 6).

Went Off the Diet   Everyone makes mistakes! But you won't suffer instant, ruinous weight gain if you slip up now and then. In fact, once you have begun to lower your setpoint, you will find that slips are easy to overcome. As Juanita Rivas puts it, "I used to panic when I went off other diets. If I gained a pound or two I figured it was all over. Now I don't even worry about it. I just keep exercising and going back to portion control." Juanita has found, and you will, too, that by returning to the plan you will resume steady, gradual weight loss.

Skipped Exercise   Skipping exercise occasionally will not hurt you—but if you let it become a habit, it can destroy all that you have worked to achieve and let your setpoint begin to inch back up to its former level.

Remember, in order to lower your setpoint, you need to exercise for 30 consecutive minutes seven days a week.

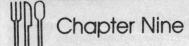 Chapter Nine

# Setpoint for Teenagers

## Can I Diet Safely in My Teen Years?

There is a Setpoint Diet for teenagers. But let me say up front that it's not for all teenagers. Younger ones still in their prime growth years, for example, should not go on a weight-loss diet without first consulting their doctor.

This may surprise you if you're an overweight teenager; after all, you are probably eager to begin shedding some pounds. But you should be aware that numerous studies have shown that younger people have different nutritional needs from adults—including a need for more calories. So what, you may wonder; if you are overweight, can't you get all the calories you need from stored fat? Unfortunately, it's not that simple.

Studies show that during your "growth spurt," which varies in age from individual to individual, the following things happen. First, your body mass actually doubles. Second, your calorie and protein requirements become higher than they will be at almost any other time of your life. And third, you become more sensitive to calorie restriction than adults. Going on a low-calorie diet at this time can interfere with that dynamic growth process, affecting your development and perhaps literally stunting your growth. As a result, most experts recommend against trying to lose weight until after you have finished your growth spurt.

There is certainly nothing wrong with following Setpoint principles—eating in balance, variety, and moderation, and exercising—but you must not even consider cutting your calories without a doctor's close supervision while you are still growing.

How can you tell when your growth spurt is over? For most girls, it is nearly completed by age 15; for boys, by 16. Therefore, you should not begin to diet except under a doctor's supervision until you reach that age—and not even then if it's obvious that your growth spurt is continuing.

Once you complete your growth spurt, you can consider starting on the special Setpoint Diet for teenagers. Because you will continue to grow (though more slowly) for a few more years, this variation of the diet allows more calories than the adult plan. Not until you reach the age of 19 will it be safe for you to go on the regular adult Setpoint plan.

## How Do I Know If I Need to Diet?

This is not so simple a question as it appears. Several factors are involved. First, you may just *feel* that you're overweight because you are larger than many of your friends; but you may simply be a "big" person, with a larger bone structure or bigger muscles than your friends. Also, being heavier than average may run in your family— do your close relatives tend to be heavyset? If so, your size may be normal for you. In that case, you should recognize that you're *never* going to look tiny; if you're preoccupied with your weight, you may be worrying unnecessarily.

Or you may be concerned because of a seemingly sudden appearance of fat on your body where there was none before. If you are in your early teens, this extra fat will probably disappear when you enter your growth-spurt years. If you are a girl, you may be concerned by new fat deposits at the hips and breasts, but these are also normal. Women generally have more fat than men; these fat deposits give your body the contours that make you look feminine.

Be sure before you consider a weight-loss diet that you really do need to lose weight. It's important that you get some professional advice on this at any age during adolescence—from your family doctor, school nurse, or health clinic. It is not uncommon for people to have distorted images of their own bodies—thinking that they are overweight when in fact they are at the weight that is right for them. This is true for many of us, because of the current unrealistic standards of thinness reflected on television and in ads. Because these superthin individuals are often actors and models whom we admire, there is a temptation to equate their leanness with worthiness. Don't fall into that trap; remember that you are a unique individual, and you shouldn't have to compete with an unrealistic ideal to demonstrate your own self-worth.

To be sure that you are not unduly influenced by media messages, ask yourself why you're concerned about losing weight. Do you hope it will make you more popular? Let you fit into clothes that are more stylish? Make you be more in control of things? If the answer to any of these questions is yes, be cautious about beginning any kind of weight-reduction program. It is true that losing weight might improve your appearance, but a slimmer body won't mean instant popularity. The most important reason to go on a diet is to improve your general well-being, and the Setpoint Diet can help you do this. But you should not expect that losing weight on this or any other diet will automatically solve any other problems you may have.

If you still feel that you need to lose weight, get professional advice in determining your desirable weight. A health professional will be able to evaluate excess body fat and determine if, and how much, you need to lose. And remember, if you are a girl 14 or under or a boy 15 or under, you should attempt to lose weight only under a doctor's supervision.

# Setpoint for Healthy Eating

Even if you decide that you shouldn't or don't want to lose weight now, you won't go wrong by adopting Setpoint principles. They are good not only for weight loss but also for a lifetime of healthy (and delicious) eating.

## Setpoint Principles

The Setpoint Diet for teenagers—like the adult plan—is based on balance, variety, and moderation in eating, combined with moderate daily exercises. Both parts of the program must be followed for success. The eating plan, unlike many extreme fad diets, ensures that you get the nutrients that your body needs at this crucial stage of your life. Among the benefits of good nutrition: good stamina, a healthy glow, a zestful manner. The exercise plan is also important, and for a number of reasons:

◊ Studies show that daily moderate exercise is essential to lower your "weight setpoint," which is the weight that your body tries to maintain no matter what you eat. If you diet without exercising, you may lose weight for a while—but eventually you'll put the weight back on.

◊ Daily moderate exercise actually *reduces* your appetite and at the same time helps you to burn calories at a higher rate throughout the day, even when you are resting.

◊ Exercise tones your body, making it firmer and more attractive, and also provides psychological benefits—helping you to relax and feel more self-confident.

For further information on the relationship between exercise and diet, read chapters 2 and 3.

Studies show that overweight teens are much more likely than their thinner counterparts to be extremely inactive—sitting when others might stand, driving the car when others would walk, taking the elevator rather than the stairs. Does this sound like you? If so, then Setpoint exercise will probably make a big difference in your life. Even if you have never thought of yourself as athletic, you will be surprised how many activities and sports you can take part in. And remember the importance of exercise: dieting alone cannot lower your setpoint and keep weight off—to do that, only moderate, daily exercise will work. If you decide to follow the Setpoint portion-control plan alone without exercise, it is highly unlikely that you will be able to keep any lost weight off for good.

# Difference between the Setpoint Diet for Teens and the Adult Setpoint Plan

Like the adult Setpoint Diet, the teen version emphasizes balance, variety, and moderation. It allows you to eat a wide variety of foods in moderate portions, balanced so that you will get the nutrients you need.

Setpoint for teens provides somewhat higher calorie and protein levels than Setpoint for adults (because you need them for continued growth). This will allow you to lose 1 to 1½ pounds every week. Losing more rapidly can be dangerous; it can mean that you are losing only water or muscle mass instead of fat. It also can mean you're not getting the nutrients you need.

The diet meets or exceeds the Recommended Dietary Allowance of nutrients for your age group. Special attention is paid to your increased requirements for protein, calcium, phosphorus, and some of the B vitamins. It is extremely flexible, to match your busy life-style—allowing you to eat a wide variety of foods, including snacks, restaurant foods, and party dishes.

# How to Go on the Setpoint Diet

Read pages 106-114 for guidelines on how to follow the Setpoint Diet for adults. Be sure you understand how the Food Group lists work and how to use portion control. Then turn back to this chapter and follow these steps:

Step One   Determine your desirable weight. Be sure to get professional advice.

Step Two   Set a realistic weight-loss schedule. Remember, this is not a "miracle" diet that promises overnight results.

Step Three   Calculate your daily calorie needs, using one of the following formulas:

**For girls,** desired weight × 12 = daily calories to start plan;

**For boys,** desired weight × 14 = daily calories to start plan.

For example, a girl with a weight goal of 123 pounds would multiply by 12 and get 1476 calories. A boy with a goal of 155 would multiply by 14 with a result of 2170.

These formulas apply until you are 22, even though you'll start using the adult portion-control plan at age 19.

Step Four   Choose the eating plan closest to the calorie level you need, using the chart on page 100 if you're under 19 or page 46 (the adult plan) if you're 19 or older. If you calculated 1572, for example, choose the 1500-calorie diet. On pages 101–105 are sample portion control charts to record your food group portions as you eat them: Make several copies and carry one with you every day.

If your calculation totals fewer than 1500 calories, choose the 1500-calorie plan anyway. As long as you exercise daily, this should lead to your weight-loss goal. It is usually not safe for teens to follow a diet of fewer than 1500 calories except under a doctor's supervision. Any diet that is so restricted in calories is certain to be deficient in nutrients as well. When you reach the age of 19, however, you may move to the adult 1200-calorie eating plan.

Step Five   Begin the Setpoint eating and exercise plan.

# Setpoint Exercise for Teens

Please read the guidelines for exercise for adults on pages 58–72. Your exercise plan will be based on the same principles. The chief difference is that you may have to be more active than the adult program requires.

There's a good reason for this: the Setpoint weight-loss plan for teens cannot depend as heavily on calorie reduction as the adult plan does, since young people must be specially concerned about getting enough of the right foods every day to support growth during these crucial years. This is why the Setpoint calorie levels for teens (page 100) are generally higher than the levels for adults (page 46). Since you will be making a more modest reduction in calories, you will have to rely more heavily on the exercise component of the Setpoint Diet to attain your weight goal.

Like the adult Setpointers, you will be choosing activities like those on the A and B lists on page 61. You'll be doing 30 consecutive minutes per day of A activities five days a week; do 30 consecutive minutes of lighter B activities on each of the other two days.

The A activities are the core of any Setpoint exercise program, for they are the key to lowering your setpoint. They are the aerobic activities, which exercise your heart and lungs—vigorous activities that use the large muscles in your body, that raise your heart rate and can make you perspire. You can add school sports such as hockey, football, and soccer to the A list.

The B exercise list contains items that are less strenuous, encompassing a wide range of recreational and leisure activities. They will not by themselves be sufficient to lower your setpoint, but they are still an important part of your overall program.

Start your exercise regimen by following the same steps covered in chapter 6. Start out slowly; don't rush it. And—if you are unathletic or self-conscious about exercising—don't despair! Just try going for a brisk walk every day; walking is an excellent way to help you get started.

How much exercise is enough? Initially you should aim for 30 minutes per day. But teenage Setpointers may need more—remember that you have to depend more on exercise than adult Setpointers do. Monitor your progress, and don't be afraid to experiment: you may find that you'll need to increase your exercise level beyond 30 minutes per day. If so, do it gradually until you determine the amount that's right for you.

In addition to your A and B exercise, you can probably benefit from trying to put more "oomph" into your daily routine activities, those things that we usually don't characterize as exercise. Remember that overweight people are often much less active than others. If you're overweight, chances are that you could profit by making some minor changes in your daily routine. You would be amazed how easy it is to put just a little more activity into your life. Consider how active you are now. Do you always take the easy way? Use the stairs; walk rather than ride; stand rather than sit. Dance more at parties. Try walking (or biking) to school, to a friend's house, or to the store. Yard work is also an excellent activity—particularly those jobs that allow you to move continuously, such as mowing the lawn with a manual mower, raking leaves, or shoveling snow. (If you enjoy these activities, you might want to start a yard service in your neighborhood—earn money while losing weight!)

## Sticking with the Setpoint Diet

Read through the tips for sticking with the Setpoint Diet in chapter 8. Pay special attention to the tips for behavior modification. You may find these techniques useful.

## Do's and Don'ts for Successful Setpointing

DO practice the Setpoint principles of balance, variety, and moderation.

DO keep a food portion record every day. Don't forget to record all snacks as you eat them.

DO add activity to your life whenever you can: walk or bike, don't drive; stand rather than sit.

DO be sure to eat a wide variety of foods. Don't have the same foods for lunch every day; try something new.

DO eat slowly, putting down your fork after each bite and chewing slowly to appreciate the taste of the food.

DON'T watch TV or read while you are eating; it's too easy to overeat if your attention is elsewhere.

DON'T try "miracle" cures for being overweight; only exercise and a well-planned, balanced diet allow you to lose weight safely and keep it off.

DON'T GO ON A CALORIE-RESTRICTED DIET IF—

◊ you are still growing rapidly, no matter what your age

◊ you have just begun to menstruate

◊ you are pregnant

◊ you are not overweight

◊ you are not sure of your reasons for wanting to diet

Talk to a doctor or counselor to make sure you really need to lose weight.

DON'T continue to lose weight once you have reached your weight goal. Read chapter 12 on Maintenance.

## Setpoint in a Social Setting

One reason some teenagers find it hard to diet is that food is a part of many social activities. But because the Setpoint Diet allows you to eat a certain amount of any food you want, this should not be a problem. For example, if you know you will be going out for pizza, remember to save the correct number of portions on your daily record (1 large slice of cheese pizza = 1 Breads/Cereals/Starchy Foods, 1 Vegetables, ½ Milk/Dairy Products, 1 A Bonus).

Likewise, if you are invited to a party, save some portions for the snacks you will eat. When you are the host, offer lower-calorie snacks such as a colorful platter of sliced raw vegetables. These will fill you up without blowing your entire snack allowance. If you have a knack for cooking you can even learn to make your own Setpoint meals and treats.

You will find that following Setpoint will be easier if you do it with other people. If your whole family is on the diet, you can give each other moral support and help solve problems. You might also enjoy planning and preparing some family meals, seeing that they follow Setpoint principles. If you have a friend who needs to lose weight, too, enlist her or him as a buddy. Eat lunch together and compare weight loss. Get a group together to play tennis, go hiking, or take a long bike ride or walk. Social events like dancing can be excellent exercise—and the more strenuous, the better. Studies show that if you have this sort of support it will be far easier to stick to the program and keep weight off.

Finally, allow yourself to feel good about yourself. You have every right to: by going on the Setpoint Diet you are adopting healthy eating and exercise habits that will serve you for a lifetime.

### The Setpoint Diet for Teens: Portions per Day (Girls 15–18, Boys 16–18)

|  | CALORIES | | | | |
|---|---|---|---|---|---|
|  | 1500 | 1800 | 2200 | 2400 | 2800 |
|  | Portions per Day | | | | |
| Breads/Cereals/ Starchy Foods | 5 | 5 | 5 | 5 | 5 |
| Fruits | 3 | 3 | 3 | 3 | 3 |
| Milk/Dairy Products | 4 | 4 | 4 | 4 | 4 |
| Meat/Poultry/ Fish | 2 | 3 | 3 | 3 | 3 |
| Vegetables | 3 | 3 | 3 | 3 | 3 |
| A Bonus | 2 | 5 | 8 | 8 | 9 |
| B Bonus | 1 | 1 | 2 | 3 | 5 |

## 1500 Calorie Portion Checklist for Teens

Date _____

| Breads/Cereals/ Starchy Foods | Fruits | Milk/Dairy Products | Meat/Fish/ Poultry | Vegetables | A Bonus | B Bonus |
|---|---|---|---|---|---|---|
| | | | | | | |
| | | | | | | |
| | | | | | | |
| | | | | | | |
| | | | | | | |

# 1800 Calorie Portion Checklist for Teens

Date _____

| Bread/Cereals/ Starchy Foods | Fruits | Milk/Dairy Products | Meat/Fish/ Poultry | Vegetables | A Bonus | B Bonus |
|---|---|---|---|---|---|---|
| | | | | | | |
| | | | | | | |
| | | | | | | |
| | | | | | | |
| | | | | | | |

# 2200 Calorie Portion Checklist for Teens

Date _____

| Breads/Cereals/ Starchy Foods | Fruits | Milk/Dairy Products | Meat/Fish/ Poultry | Vegetables | A Bonus | B Bonus |
|---|---|---|---|---|---|---|
| | | | | | | |
| | | | | | | |
| | | | | | | |
| | | | | | | |
| | | | | | | |
| | | | | | | |
| | | | | | | |

# 2400 Calorie Portion Checklist for Teens

Date _____

| Breads/Cereals/Starchy Foods | Fruits | Milk/Dairy Products | Meat/Fish/Poultry | Vegetables | A Bonus | B Bonus |
|---|---|---|---|---|---|---|
| | | | | | | |
| | | | | | | |
| | | | | | | |
| | | | | | | |
| | | | | | | |

## 2800 Calorie Portion Checklist for Teens

Date _____

| Breads/Cereals/Starchy Foods | Fruits | Milk/Dairy Products | Meat/Fish/Poultry | Vegetables | A Bonus | B Bonus |
|---|---|---|---|---|---|---|
| | | | | | | |
| | | | | | | |
| | | | | | | |
| | | | | | | |
| | | | | | | |
| | | | | | | |
| | | | | | | |

# Chapter Ten

# Setpoint for Older Adults

Ten percent of all Americans today are sixty-five or older, and the percentage of older people is expected to rise dramatically in coming years. At the same time, the image of old age is changing. No longer is growing older considered to be synonymous with sickness and frailty; in many cases, as you know, just the opposite is true. Jack La Lanne, the physical fitness guru who recently turned 70, possesses a body that would be the envy of a 20-year-old. Walt Stack, a legendary marathoner who lives near San Francisco, also in his seventies, runs up to 30 miles a day. The obvious health and energy of these men are dramatic proof that retirement doesn't have to mean consignment to a rocking chair.

Of course, not everyone would be interested in the rigorous regimens that Stack and La Lanne follow. But even moderate amounts of regular exercise pay dividends in health and well-being. Ronald Reagan has been active all his life, riding horses and chopping wood. He is a vivid example of the health and strength that are possible in advanced years, given a regimen of physical activity. Mr. Reagan shows little evidence of his age.

It is not a coincidence that these three men are physically active and that they show few signs of the inevitable declines of age. The truth is that very few of those declines are, in fact, inevitable; growing evidence indicates that many of the ailments that have been associated with old age—including stiffness, osteoporosis, even some forms of arthritis—are at least in part diseases of disuse.

Yes, exercise is important—but so is good nutrition. Everyone knows that an improper diet can have serious medical consequences. It can cause osteoporosis and iron deficiency anemia, for example. It can also lead to obesity, a prime suspect in heart disease, stroke, and adult-onset diabetes. Also you may be among that 20 percent of the American population that is susceptible to hypertension (high blood pressure)—too much sodium is one of several factors that can promote this disorder.

The best way to avoid many of these so-called "problems of aging" seems to be through a regimen of healthy eating and exercise. Adopting such a plan at any age can only enhance the quality of your life, no matter what your present age or condition. And just as there is evidence that physical activity and good nutrition can prevent problems from occurring, there is growing evidence that the opposite may also be the case: that poor nutrition and inactivity can cause or exacerbate problems, including some mental and emotional problems that have often been incorrectly ascribed to "senility."

The Setpoint plan for older adults is designed to encourage both physical activity *and* good nutrition. It makes it easy and pleasant for you to lose weight—or maintain your present weight—while eating a balanced, nutritious diet, and to add as much healthful activity as is possible to your life.

## Confronting—and Overcoming— Obstacles

Let's face it—some older Americans have to confront problems that may not afflict other segments of our population. These may make it more difficult to get the exercise and good nutrition you need.

The good news is that most—if not all—such problems can be overcome. The first challenge is to take a hard look at your own situation and confront your problems squarely; the second is to resolve to do all you can to meet them.

Let's look at a few examples. Some older people experience a decline in their ability to taste and smell; the obvious result is that food doesn't seem as appetizing as it once did. A problem, yes. But unsolvable? Of course not. You can spice up your food or include in your diet those foods that have a stronger taste and aroma. Experiment, especially with sauces.

Many people—young and old alike—don't relish eating alone; they think the effort of food preparation may not be "worth it." If you're one of those people, *do* something about it! Invite in a friend, or alternate cooking responsibilities with a neighbor. If there is a senior citizens center nearby, take advantage of any meal services it offers. Remember that eating should be fun, and living alone absolutely should not be allowed to ruin the enjoyment—and good nutrition—you get from eating well-balanced meals.

There are other food-related difficulties that older people may experience; again, all can be compensated for. Some adults of all ages, for example, lose their ability to digest milk, a key source of protein and calcium. Others experience a natural reduction in the amount of acid in the stomach, so it becomes more difficult to digest meat—a good source of protein. Some people find raw vegetables and fruit difficult to chew; this can cause vitamin deficiencies and constipation due to lack of fiber.

These deficiencies *can* be remedied, in most cases fairly simply, by following a healthy, balanced diet. If one type of food presents a problem, there's always another that can take its place. The Setpoint Diet, with its emphasis on balance, variety, and moderation, is ideal. The diet itself, as you know, is scientifically designed to make sure that you get the ideal number of servings from each food group each day. The emphasis on variety assures that you get the nutrients you need at the same time. Variety is especially important for older people: by consciously selecting many different foods, you can prevent boredom that causes so many to simply lose their appetites.

## Setpoint for Good Nutrition

Because your nutritional needs are different at this time of life, your lifelong habits of eating may no longer ensure that you get all the nutrients that your body requires. As you get older, the following become especially important:

Calories   Because the basal metabolic rate declines about 10 percent per decade, you need fewer calories than when you were younger. Because it is often easier to eat calorie-dense foods—such as sweets and fried foods—you may actually be consuming more calories than you need while at the same time becoming deficient in some vitamins and minerals. The Setpoint eating plan will provide you with the right number of calories while making certain that you are getting the nutrients you need.

Protein   Your body needs protein to rebuild muscle tissue and to form enzymes, which keep the body functioning properly. Meat and milk are good sources; so are poultry, fish, eggs, beans, cheese, nuts, and soybean products, such as tofu (soybean curd).

Calcium   Adequate calcium, which is essential for strong bones and teeth, is especially important for older adults. It is now known that osteoporosis, or "brittle bones," results from a combination of inactivity and inadequate calcium intake. Women, who are particularly prone to this disorder, should consciously increase the amount of calcium that they eat throughout life. The best sources of calcium include all dairy products—especially milk, yogurt, and cheese—and fish canned with the bones, such as salmon and sardines. Dark green leafy vegetables such as collards and spinach are also good sources, but their calcium may not be as readily absorbed by the body. Note that calcium is absorbed readily only in the presence of vitamin D. Make sure that you get plenty of sunshine, which allows your skin to manufacture this vitamin, or drink vitamin D–fortified milk.

Zinc   Zinc, which is important for proper healing as well as for vision, is often deficient in older people's diets. The best sources of zinc are oysters, beef, veal, lamb, pork, organ meats, turkey, and eggs. Other important sources include fish, cheese (cheddar and mozzarella), chicken, and legumes (lentils, chick peas, and pinto beans). Although portions are generally small, wheat germ and nuts are also sources of zinc. Many ready-to-eat cereals are fortified with zinc; check labels for zinc levels.

Iron   Iron, which is an important constituent of your blood, is available in a wide variety of foods. Best sources include organ meats, beef, veal, lamb, and eggs. Other sources include the dark meat of turkey, legumes, enriched bread products, and the ready-to-eat cereals that are fortified with iron.

Fiber   As I mentioned, lack of fiber can cause constipation. Recent research indicates that the various forms of fiber perform far more functions than simply the regulation of bowel movements: there is some evidence that adequate fiber can help reduce cholesterol and may even act as a protective factor against some cancers. Good sources of fiber include whole grain or bran cereals and breads, fruits and vegetables, nuts and seeds.

Because it may be difficult to eat some of these foods, many people don't get nearly enough fiber. It is important to try to find a solution that suits your own needs and life-style. You can, for example, select ready-to-eat cereals high in fiber. If you have severe problems with chewing, eat fruits and vegetables pureed—they will taste just as good, and the fiber is still available. Don't try to get all your fiber from one kind of food. If you are not currently eating high-fiber foods, add them gradually to your diet.

Fluids   For optimum functioning, your body requires an adequate amount of fluids. Many Americans, including older citizens, do not drink enough liquids; this can cause or exacerbate such problems as indigestion and constipation. Whether you get it through water, milk, fruit juice, or soda, try to consume a minimum of three to five cups of fluid every single day.

Sodium   Sodium is not a problem for most people. But it can contribute to hypertension among the 20 percent of the population that is susceptible to this disease. Following a low-sodium diet requires learning to eat foods without added salt and to avoid foods with high salt content. Use the salt shaker sparingly, and then only after tasting the foods. Read food labels to determine sodium content. Use less salt in cooking; use other seasonings instead.

You may find it easiest to cut down on salt gradually, over a period of days or weeks. As many people who have gone on low-sodium diets will tell you, after a time you will no longer miss salt (which is an acquired taste) and may, in fact, find that foods taste better than ever before, especially when flavored with herbs, spices, or lemon juice.

# Setpoint for Older People: Dieting

It may not be necessary or appropriate to go on a calorie-reduced diet if you are over 80, although following Setpoint principles can be an excellent way of improving your overall nutrition and physical fitness.

For overweight people under 80, the Setpoint Diet does provide a safe and well-balanced plan for gradual, steady weight loss. One reason that so many of us become overweight in old age is that while our basal metabolic rate is declining, so is our level of activity. Lean body mass (muscle) is reduced; fat becomes more noticeable. For some reason, age-related obesity appears to be more prevalent in women than in men. Again, a big contributor to this weight gain is that combination of poor nutrition and lack of activity.

Obesity at any age can cause a number of psychological and other health problems: in older adults especially it may worsen any preexisting health problems, such as cardiac, joint, and pulmonary disorders. Also, the extra weight makes it even harder to move about, thus making exercise—and, in some cases, even self-care—difficult. And, of course, weighing more than the ideal can contribute to a lowering of self-image, thus exacerbating any feelings of depression or loneliness.

To follow the Setpoint program for weight loss, read through the guidelines in chapter 5 on how to follow the program. Then begin, giving special attention to the nutrients listed above. Some women may find it necessary to eat fewer than 1200 calories daily in order to lose weight. If you don't lose on Setpoint's 1200-calorie level, ask your doctor to help you adapt the plan to your needs. Such a restricted diet may not supply the nutrients you need, so be sure to take a supplement. The kind to look for is one that includes a broad range of vitamins and minerals. Stay away from products that give you more than 100 percent of the U.S. Recommended Daily Allowances; these are a waste of money, and overdoses of some vitamins can be dangerous.

## Setpoint Exercise for Older People

Why Exercise at My Age?   Although exercise is important at any age, it can make a very big difference in the lives of people who are growing older. Not only does exercise help to prevent many of the ailments of old age we have been talking about, but it can also help to ease preexisting conditions. It can improve the condition of your heart and circulatory system; it can prevent or cure insomnia; it relieves stress and helps ease depression; it speeds the intestinal transit time of food, helping to alleviate constipation; it retards the normal, age-related replacement of muscle with fat; it helps to retard osteoporosis in women; and, of course, it helps to control excess weight and thus leads to improved appearance and self-esteem.

With all of these benefits, it seems surprising that the gyms and parks are not crowded with exercising older people—but, alas, such is not the case. In many instances they may not have thought that much about the many benefits of exercise. In all too many other cases, however, they are reluctant to do so because it may not appear seemly or appropriate for their age.

This is absolute nonsense. If you have been harboring fears about what people may think of you if you join an exercise class or begin a walking program, put those fears right out of your head. I can assure you that the majority of people will think that what you are doing is *terrific* and will even applaud you. Some of the loudest cheers at the New York Marathon every year come for the older runners, some in their eighties, who are performing a feat—running 26 miles—that the vast majority of men and women in their twenties and thirties cannot do.

Even if you have never been athletic, you can begin some sort of exercise activity right now. I can promise you that if you do so and keep it up it will enhance your life. As Jack La Lanne says, "I really don't give a damn how long I live, but I want to live while I'm living."

How to Exercise    The ideal situation for any older adult is to be able to continue the vigorous exercise you have been performing your whole life. I realize that for many this is impossible and that a number of older people are inactive. Many have been very inactive for some period of time, perhaps years.

However, the good news is that you can begin some form of physical activity at any age and that it will pay enormous dividends in terms of health and well-being.

The following discussion of exercise should be taken as a guideline only. The exercise needs and capabilities of older Americans vary enormously, ranging from the superfit, like Walt Stack, to many who, because of reduced mobility, are virtually chairbound.

If you are like many older people, you can follow the regular Setpoint exercise plan (see chapter 6). Activities

such as walking, bicycling, swimming—even jogging—
are performed daily by countless older Americans. It is
possible and desirable to try to achieve aerobic fitness,
even if you have never exercised before. The main caveats
are to see a doctor before you begin and to start out slowly
and not try to achieve too much too rapidly. If you are
able to perform these types of activity, you will quickly
reach your weight goal and be rewarded with a sense of
well-being you may not have felt for years, if ever!

If, on the other hand, your mobility is impaired because
of joint problems or heart disease, you can still begin to
add exercise and movement to your life. One place to
begin is to try stretching more. The first thing when you
wake up, take a few minutes and stretch all of the muscles
in your body, then relax. Try to set aside 10 minutes twice
a day to perform more stretches. You will be surprised
how quickly this will improve your limberness and even
chase away aches and pains.

Apart from stretching, simply try to put more movement into your life. Stand instead of sit, for example; try
to walk more rather than driving; do gardening or anything
else you enjoy. Stretch while you're watching TV. Or take
up some kind of sport that is fun for you—maybe something you have always wanted to try.

Finally, no matter what your condition, one of the best
things I can advise you to do is to join a fitness center
that offers programs for older citizens. There you will be
able to adopt a regimen that's tailored to your individual
needs—many older people have discovered yoga, for
example, as a way of regaining the suppleness of youth
(stiffness, as with many other disorders, is largely an ail-
ment of disuse). Not only does the exercise make you
feel good, but the social setting of any exercise class can
provide special opportunities that may open up whole new
horizons!

# Chapter Eleven

# Questions People Ask about the Setpoint Diet

*How can I measure my setpoint?*

Your setpoint can't be read the way body temperature can. It isn't a static number engraved on your brain—rather, it's a range of two or three pounds within which your body tries to maintain your weight. It can change in the course of your life. Your setpoint is the weight that you maintain when you don't pay conscious attention to what you are eating.

*Why does my husband lose weight faster than I do?*

Many things in life aren't "fair," and one of them is that men lose weight on Setpoint more rapidly than women! There are two main reasons for this. First, he probably weighs a great deal more than you do, and the heavier you are the more quickly you will lose weight. Second, he probably has a higher ratio of muscle to total body weight. Muscle, you'll recall, is more metabolically active than fat, so a larger percentage of his body can burn calories for energy.

*What happens if I miss a day of exercise?*

If it's only one day, nothing will happen. But if you allow yourself to begin exercising irregularly, the benefits of *regular* exercise—including the lowering of your setpoint—will disappear. Remember that for the exercise plan to be effective you must exercise continuously for a half hour a day.

*I never had trouble with my weight until after I had a baby. I just can't seem to shake that extra 15 pounds.*

Unfortunately, this is a common experience; many women find it very hard to maintain a desirable weight after pregnancy. It appears that pregnancy itself raises the setpoint—and it doesn't always return to pre-pregnancy levels! Fortunately, regular exercise can offset this rise. Engaging in some form of exercise during pregnancy—under your doctor's supervision, of course—may help you recover more quickly after the baby is born. If you follow the diet and exercise components of Setpoint after your baby is born, your weight should soon be back to prepregnancy levels.

*I'm not really overweight—I just have too much fat on my hips. Is there some specific exercise for taking that off?*

Despite flim-flam advertising for miracle wraps and spot-reducing machines, there is no way to take fat off one selected place on the body. Combining the Setpoint Diet with the exercise plan should help you to lose excess fat all over your body while firming your thighs.

*Following a diet seems like too much trouble. What about diet pills and diet candies?*

Diet candies are a waste of money; there is absolutely no evidence that they work. It's possible that eating a candy before a meal might cut your appetite somewhat, but if you don't lower your setpoint you will not be able to keep weight off.

As for diet pills, they are potent, potentially dangerous drugs. It is true that they work in some people to suppress the appetite, but as soon as you quit taking them your appetite will return and your weight will also return to your setpoint level. Because of their possible side effects—nervousness, insomnia, elevated blood pressure—diet pills are not safe to take for long periods of time.

Obviously, the best way to lose weight is to adopt a healthy life-style. Eat right and get the exercise you need.

*I've always been fairly active. I started the Setpoint Diet, but when I go for a walk I can't get my pulse above 100— no matter how fast I walk. Is the diet working for me?*

Everybody is different. A fit individual may need to perform an exercise more vigorous than walking to ensure raising the pulse rate into the target zone. Walking will undoubtedly be enough to keep your setpoint from creeping upward, but in your case it is probably not enough, in itself, to lower it.

*Must I eat all the portions listed in the diet?*

Yes. To ensure balanced nutrition, you must eat all the portions specified from the major food groups: Bread/Cereals/Starchy Foods, Fruits, Milk/Dairy Products, Meat/Poultry/Fish and Vegetables. In addition, to ensure an adequate caloric intake, you should eat either all the Bonus servings listed for your calorie level or, if you prefer, substitute more portions from the regular food groups. Look at the "Or Substitute" sections at the bottom of the Bonus lists to see what you may substitute.

*Will my appetite increase if I exercise?*

Remember that regular, moderate exercise itself is a proven appetite depressant; it both lowers your setpoint and reduces your appetite. When you stop regular exercise, your appetite and your setpoint will begin to creep up to their former levels.

*I do plenty of strenuous work around the house. Why doesn't that count?*

Housework and yardwork are excellent for burning calories. And it's true that such exercise may be vigorous enough to elevate your heart rate. Still, most work around the house is not performed continuously.

You *must* exercise continuously, at your target heart rate, for 30 minutes to affect your setpoint.

*Are there combinations of food particularly good for burning fat or building muscle?*

This is a tempting idea. However, there is no evidence that any combinations of food work to cause your body selectively to burn fat. As I explained earlier, fat is used only when your body needs it for energy. As for certain foods that are reported to build muscle selectively, that, too, is a myth. Your muscles are largely made up of the constituents of proteins, but eating a great deal of protein will not result in more muscle—instead, the excess will be stored as fat. For a reduction of body fat and an increase in muscle tissue, exercise and follow the portion-control plan, which gives you the nutrients you need in balanced proportions.

*How much alcohol can I drink on this diet? My bonuses seem to allow quite a lot.*

The Bonus lists are designed to help you add variety and enjoyment to your diet. But—just as you should vary the foods you eat within each food group—you should not use all your Bonuses on alcohol!

Remember the key words: balance, variety, and moderation. With alcoholic beverages in particular, moderation is the best policy.

*What if I follow the diet but don't exercise?*

You will lose weight for a while, and you will certainly be on a balanced, nutritious diet. But remember that diet alone won't change your setpoint. Thus, your appetite will not decrease, so you will probably be hungry most of the time.

Experience also shows that most people in that situation will reach a weight-loss plateau, get discouraged, go off the diet, and soon regain what they have lost. I wrote this book to help people get out of that sad routine once and for all.

*What about junk food on the diet?*

There is *no such thing* as junk food! That's because *any* food, eaten in moderation, can fit into a well-balanced diet. There are no "bad" foods; similarly, there are no "perfect" foods.

However, there can certainly be junk *diets!* The important thing is to consume the nutrients our bodies need in the proper proportion. Every one of us can do that by observing the cornerstones of good nutrition: balance, variety, and moderation.

If you remember these three magic words, you can eat right—and you can do so enjoyably and within any budget.

*I'd like to give up smoking, but I'm afraid I'll gain weight.*

It's good that you recognize the health risks of smoking and want to give it up. Nicotine does lower the setpoint, and this appears to be a major reason for weight gain upon quitting. Thus, following the Setpoint Diet can be essential to the success of your antismoking program. Not only will it counter the rise in setpoint spurred by nicotine withdrawal, but the effect of appetite reduction also should help keep you from overeating. Whenever you find yourself craving a cigarette, performing some physical activity may help—taking a brisk walk, for example. Because the diet itself is so varied and liberal, you will be able to "reward" yourself several times a day with a healthy, tasty snack—instead of a smoke. As a bonus, your daily exercise should help you feel far less nervous as you go through withdrawal pangs.

*Why does it get harder to keep weight off as I get older?*

I mentioned earlier that our basal metabolic rate declines about 10 percent per decade. Thus, if you don't compensate for that decrease by eating less or exercising more, you will inevitably gain weight.

Fortunately, the daily exercise you get on the Setpoint Diet will lower your setpoint and make up for any age-induced decline of basal metabolic rate.

*Can I use the Setpoint Diet to gain weight?*

Yes! The Setpoint Diet is designed to be a healthy, lifelong eating plan, and its principles apply whether you want to lose, maintain—or gain—weight. Underweight people should use the standard procedure for getting started on the Setpoint Diet. They would no doubt start on a higher-calorie plan and they might have to increase portion sizes or numbers.

Many very thin people have poor, unbalanced diets. They may not even enjoy their food, so they may not eat enough to get balanced nutrition. If this is your problem, going on the Setpoint Diet should greatly improve the balance of your diet. Perhaps your appetite will also improve as you begin to eat healthfully.

*Why can't I lose weight more rapidly on the Setpoint Diet?*

Although 1–3 pounds a week may *seem* slow, it is actually an optimal rate for weight loss. A faster loss indicates that you are probably losing water and lean body mass—not fat. It's true that many "fad" diets promise spectacular results; it's also true that they just don't work over the long term.

*Is it all right to exercise when I'm sick?*

If you have a mild cold or simply feel out of sorts, exercise may actually make you feel better. However, if you are really sick—are running a fever or have sore, swollen glands—it's better to stay in bed and give your body a rest. A good rule of thumb is that if you are too sick to go to work, you shouldn't exercise.

## Chapter Twelve

# Setpoint for a Lifetime

"This is the first diet I ever went on without an automatic penalty at the end," says Chuck Roberts, who has lost 68 pounds on the Setpoint Diet. "On all the other diets, you can lose weight all right—but as soon as you finish, it comes right back on, much faster than you lost it. With Setpoint it stays off."

"It's a very forgiving diet," echoes Melba Luongo, who lost 12 pounds. "If you slip, you don't immediately regain ten pounds like on other diets."

As you know, the Setpoint Diet works so well and continues to work because it changes your setpoint. When Chuck, who has described himself as a "professional dieter," went off any other diet, of course he gained weight quickly—because his body marshaled all its resources to return him to his former weight. Likewise, when Melba "cheated" on ordinary diets, her body quickly converted the excess calories into fat—its response to the "starving" reflex brought on by her reduced-calorie intake. Now, with a lower Setpoint, if she overindulges occasionally, her weight changes little if at all. Her body is now more efficient at "wasting" excess calories.

Furthermore, both Chuck and Melba say, as do so many other Setpointers, that the temptation to binge occurs less frequently now. That's because the diet has normalized their appetite-control mechanism.

# Why the Setpoint Diet Is for a Lifetime

The reason that so many dieters find themselves caught in the yo-yo syndrome—losing and then regaining weight, bouncing from one diet to another—is that other diets not only fail to lower the setpoint, but many of them are unbalanced (especially those that emphasize only a few foods). Such a diet is not healthy and can be dangerous.

Learning to eat according to Setpoint principles changes your eating habits so that once you lose pounds, you can maintain your lower weight through a lifetime of healthy eating and exercise. Because the Setpoint Diet is balanced to provide the nutrients you need, it is an eating plan that you can follow for a lifetime.

# Maintenance—Living with Setpoint

Weight maintenance on the Setpoint Diet is easy. You just continue to exercise and to practice portion control. Of course, it will be a lot easier once you have reached your target weight! At that point you can add more food to your daily menu. Here's how it works.

1. Exercise Maintenance   With any exercise program, the hardest part is beginning; maintenance is easy. Continue to exercise for one-half hour daily, but if you want, you can reduce the number of days you do A exercises to three or four per week. This will be sufficient to maintain aerobic fitness and keep your setpoint at its new, lower level. Three times per week is a minimum, however. Anything less and you will lose your aerobic fitness and your weight will begin to creep up. On remaining days of the week, engage in B activities.

If you begin to gain weight, return to five days of A exercise and/or increase the intensity of your exercise. Check your pulse to be sure you are in the target zone. Consider your diet also—it may be necessary to return to a lower-calorie–level Setpoint plan, as discussed below.

2. Diet maintenance    The second step in maintaining your new weight is to increase your calorie intake about 300 calories. Note that this may mean merely switching to the next-higher calorie level of the Setpoint Diet. In any event, keep on eating the Setpoint way.

Now monitor your weight for two weeks: if it stays steady, you'll know you have arrived at the right calorie intake for you. If you continue losing, add another 300 calories to your daily intake. If you continue to lose even on the 2400-calorie plan, continue to increase every few weeks in increments of 300 calories (equivalent to 1 B Bonus plus 2 A Bonuses). With experimentation, you should soon determine the right calorie level for you.

If, on the other hand, you begin gaining weight again, return to the lower-calorie eating plan or increase the intensity of your exercise if you can do so without over-doing it. Try jogging, say, instead of walking, or pedaling faster on the exercise bike (but always within your target heart zone).

The important thing is not to make too many changes too quickly. Give your body time to adapt. Ultimately, as long as you continue to exercise daily or nearly so and you continue to practice portion control, you should reach a balance of diet and exercise that will maintain you at your ideal weight indefinitely.

# Maintenance Tips

◊ You will probably find, as have many Setpointers, that after several weeks or months on the diet, you will automatically adjust and compensate for temporary changes in your life-style—such as going on vacation or occasionally overeating during the holidays (see pp. 128–129 for tips on handling holiday eating).

◊ To anticipate some fluctuations in your weight and at the same time to make sure that you don't gradually gain without realizing it, it is a good idea to set an acceptable weight range for yourself (a 5-pound range, perhaps, such as 125 to 130 pounds). Monitor your weight by continuing to weigh yourself once a week at about the same time.

◊ If you find it necessary to return to a lower-calorie level, go back to the things you did that were helpful when you first began the Setpoint plan. Back then you were probably keeping portion control records, preplanning your daily menus, and weighing and measuring your foods. If these things worked once, they'll work again.

◊ Sometimes it is difficult to maintain your new weight because you may have trouble accepting the image of your new slimmer body! To help overcome this, buy yourself a new outfit that makes you feel and look good at your new weight. (Many formerly heavy dieters unthinkingly continue to buy and wear clothes that are too large for their new weight.) Likewise, don't keep your "fat clothes" tucked in the back of the closet "just in case." Have them altered to fit your new self, or give them to charity. As long as you continue to follow Setpoint principles, you will never need those baggy clothes again.

## Making the Diet a Part of Your Life

Setpoint in a Family Setting   As we saw in chapter 7, "Adopting Setpoint Smoothly," your family can be a big help to you if they follow Setpoint, too. Of course, they will be helping themselves as well by exercising and by eating healthfully. If you have children, discuss the diet with them and let them help plan menus. Susan Philbrick explained Setpoint to her children, ages three and six, and found it "an excellent tool for teaching nutrition!" By impressing on children the principles of balance, variety, and moderation, you will be helping to start them on a lifetime of healthy living.

Encourage the whole family to experiment with new foods, which is an easy way to get more variety into your diet. Make family dinners an event: use your good china and serve food as attractively as possible. Don't think of Setpoint food as "diet food"—which it isn't.

Finally, continue to encourage your family to exercise with you. Take your kids when you go for a walk or jog; stage informal competitions on the exercise bike; play basketball or badminton; go bowling together. Not only will you help your children develop a lifelong love for activity; you will grow closer as a family.

An important note for parents: the Setpoint Diet is *not* intended to be a reducing plan for children, even those who may be very overweight. Children who have not yet completed their preadolescent "growth spurt" should *never* attempt to lose weight, except under a physician's close supervision. Restricting calories at this time can interfere with normal development.

Likewise, the degree of the child's obesity should be determined by a physician using skin-fold–thickness charts and growth charts and taking into consideration where on the growth curve the child is. Many cases of childhood obesity are simply outgrown; in fact, an overweight child in a family whose members are of normal weight has a high chance of becoming a normal-weight adult. An obese child in a family with one or more obese adults, however, does have a high probability of becoming an obese adult; in this event the family should work together on weight management, seeking professional help.

If you or your preadolescent child is concerned about her weight, the best thing you can do is encourage the child to become more active. Numerous studies show a close relationship between childhood obesity and inactivity. Tell her that temporary overweight is common in pre-teens and reassure her that she is likely to outgrow it. Don't nag her or make her feel self-conscious. Be constructive. Make sure she understands the importance of being active. Help her plan ways to get more exercise, perhaps through family activities.

Once a teen has finished his or her growth spurt, a modified version of the Setpoint diet, detailed in chapter 9, can be used for weight reduction and maintenance. The age at which this diet can be followed will vary: as a rule, most girls can begin to follow it at 15 and most boys by 16.

The question of dieting for teenagers is a thorny one— so much social life involves food, and adolescence is a time of volatile emotion. Therefore, it is important to approach the subject of overweight very cautiously. Bear in mind that teenagers' feelings of self-worth may be tied up in feelings about their bodies. If a teenage girl sees herself as fat, she may conclude that she is virtually "worthless." Some teens, especially girls, may become so obsessed with losing weight that they become anorexic (obsessed with thinness to the point of near-starvation) or bulimic (given to binge eating followed by self-induced vomiting). At the same time, the teenage years are a time of experimentation with independence, so your child may not be receptive to your attempts to reassure her about her body.

The two most important things you can do are first, encourage your overweight teen to get more exercise (but without seeming pushy—perhaps organize a family hiking trip once a week) and second, be positive. Don't nag or pressure the child; for adolescent dieting to be successful, the teen must be self-motivated and ready to diet.

If a teenager in your family is interested in dieting (perhaps inspired by your weight loss on Setpoint!) let him or her read chapter 9 on Setpoint for teens. If his preadolescent growth spurt is complete and he wants to try the diet, assure him that you will do everything you can to help. Reread chapter 9 yourself so you will be aware of the ways in which the special regimen for teens differs from the adult Setpoint Diet.

Bear in mind that in certain circumstances weight reduction should not be attempted except under guidance of a physician. These circumstances are: before and during the growth-spurt phase, usually in the early teens; during adolescent pregnancy; when the young person is not obese; when he or she is emotionally unsettled (even if fat); and immediately after a girl first begins to menstruate.

Eating Out    Eating in restaurants can pose a challenge: not only are you unable to control how the food is prepared, but restaurant portions are often much bigger than those you would serve at home. On traditionally restricted diets, finding something "legal" to eat in a restaurant is almost impossible; with Setpoint, you can choose literally anything on the menu, as long as you don't exceed the daily number of portions allowed per food group.

Try to maintain as much control as possible: don't be afraid to be assertive. Be very specific when placing your order. If you are unsure how a dish is prepared, by all means ask. Foods that are baked, roasted, boiled, or broiled are lower in calories than comparable foods that are fried, sautéed, or breaded. Ask for sauces and gravies on the side so you can control how much of them you eat. If something arrives that is not prepared the way you asked for it, do not hesitate to send it back. Order from the à la carte side of the menu. That way you can choose exactly the food groups that you want to eat.

Although you generally have no control over the size of portions served, you should by now have a feel for what an ounce and a cup look like. Feel free to ask for smaller portions or even children's portions. Order an appetizer in place of an entree, or try sharing your order with a companion. Remember that you don't have to be a member of the clean-plate club!

Because more restaurants are catering to dieters and health-conscious eaters, some menus now feature low-calorie specials. Also growing in popularity are salad bars. Take advantage of the salad bar by using a generous serving of spinach or lettuce as the base. Toppings and additions are allowed, but remember they must all be counted. Extra calories can add up fast—especially from cole slaw, potato salad, pasta salads, and the like together with their dressings. Go for the fresh vegetables and choose a low-calorie dressing.

When eating Chinese or Mexican food, watch the before-dinner "munchies" of noodles or nachos. It's easy to consume all your B Bonuses even before you've started your dinner. Likewise, if a basket of bread is placed on the table, don't eat too much! Ask that it be removed if its presence is too great a temptation.

For more tips on eating in restaurants, see also "A Treasury of Tips," chapter 8.

Eating at a friend's house can sometimes raise an even greater temptation than eating in a restaurant, because it may not be easy to decline a particularly rich dish. Don't be afraid to tell your friend, well before the dinner party, that you are on a diet. Ask her or him to serve you smaller portions. As with restaurant eating, maintain as much control as possible over your intake by asking for sauces and dressing on the side.

Resist temptation and don't worry about hurting your host's or hostess's feelings by not eating everything offered. Remember that anyone who insists that you go off your diet "just this once" isn't behaving like a real friend.

Coping with Holidays and Parties    Perhaps the time of greatest temptation for any dieter is during holidays and at parties. Because the Setpoint Diet allows you to eat such a wide variety of food, you needn't give up any special treat as long as you can eat it in controlled amounts. If you are invited to a party, it's a good idea to save your daily Bonus foods for snacks, drinks, or desserts. Also you might want to curb your appetite with fruit or raw vegetables before going to the party so you won't feel so tempted to munch on higher-calorie foods.

And speaking of fruits and vegetables: party givers are increasingly serving sliced raw vegetables with dips. The vegetables are delicious by themselves, so it is not necessary to use the often-rich dips provided. Likewise, while Setpoint does allow for a cocktail or two, remember that diet sodas, seltzer, and mineral water are Freebies; in these days of health consciousness you need not fear that you will be considered odd for forgoing alcoholic beverages.

Let's face it: holidays are traditionally times of overindulgence. Furthermore, you can become so busy during this period that your attention is no longer focused on diet and exercise. If I had to give just one piece of advice for coping with the temptations of the holidays, it would be first and foremost to continue to perform your A exercise five times a week. This will go a long way toward making up for any overindulgence.

Making Setpoint International    Again because it offers such a variety of food, Setpoint is easy to adapt to international and ethnic cuisine. To determine portions of ethnic favorites, simply follow the guidelines for combination foods. Thus 2 tacos count as 2 Breads/Cereals/Starchy Foods, 1½ Meat/Poultry/Fish, 1 Vegetable, ½ Milk/Dairy Products, and ½ A Bonus.

Remember also when preparing ethnic foods to emphasize Setpoint principles. While a tablespoon of sour cream may be delicious on borscht, the same amount of plain yogurt tastes nearly as good and contains about half the calories. Likewise, there are a number of low-fat sauces that can be served over pasta in place of rich, creamy sauces (try the Setpoint Pasta Primavera on p. 245). When an ingredient must be fried, cut down on the amount of oil used or cook it in a no-stick frying pan. Likewise, tortillas needn't be fried for tostados; instead, they can be wrapped in foil and heated. (See recipe for Tostados on p. 249.)

Traveling with Setpoint    Traveling, whether for business or pleasure, can challenge the most dedicated dieter. Again, Setpoint is extremely adaptable—just remember the Setpoint principles of balance, variety, and moderation. This will help you when you must eat often in restaurants or from room service.

To make sure you get enough fruit and vegetables, it might be a good idea to bring some along from home. If you are on an extended trip, try to find a deli or supermarket somewhere near your hotel where you can replenish your supply of fruit and perhaps pick up a portion of low-fat cheese for snacks in your room. Often you can order a fruit plate in restaurants, but be careful: canned (and sometimes fresh) fruits served in restaurants are often swimming in heavy syrup or drenched with sugar, thus counting as an additional A Bonus.

Likewise, you might try ordering vegetarian meals when

traveling by plane. These often consist of large salad plates, with fruits and vegetables, and sometimes a hard-boiled egg or cheese. Or pack your own lunch—nobody says you *have* to eat airline food!

One of your most important travel plans should be to continue your daily exercise. Besides keeping you on your Setpoint schedule, exercise can help you overcome jet lag and stiffness from travel. If your customary exercise is jogging, it will be especially easy: in fact, this can be a fun way to sightsee in a new place. Because so many people all over the world jog today, some hotels even provide jogging trails on the grounds. Ask the bell captain where joggers usually go; or simply carry a map of the city with you and set out. Be creative: a young woman I know who frequently travels tells me that if she cannot find another route, she simply jogs around the parking lot of her hotel or motel.

Many hotels have swimming pools, and an increasing number are installing gyms and fitness rooms. If your hotel provides such a service, by all means take advantage of it. But remember to stay active even if you can't follow your regular program exactly. A brisk walk can be a good way to get to know the town, so walk to and from restaurants when feasible instead of driving or taking a cab. On vacations, take your bicycle along, or rent one when you reach your destination.

**A Final Word**   By now I hope that you have become a dedicated Setpointer—or are at least ready to begin. If you have been following Setpoint principles for several days or weeks, you undoubtedly have already begun to experience the many benefits of portion control and exercise: weight loss, greater energy and an improved sense of well-being. Congratulations, and keep up the good work! You now know that the small amount of effort and planning you have put in are more than worth it. And remember as you continue to follow Setpoint that it is not just a diet—it is a way of life that promotes good health and good eating for a lifetime.

# Menus

The following pages promise good eating. They contain menus and recipes to make it easy for you to eat the Setpoint way.

You may use them if and as you see fit—as presented, as amended to suit your tastes, or not at all. They are not Setpoint requirements. But they can help make Setpoint easy and more enjoyable.

The menus reflect portion-counting already done for you by nutritionists at General Foods. There are 42 menus—14 geared generally to adult calorie levels and tastes, 14 with particular appeal to older adults, and 14 designed especially for adolescents.

These menus reflect differences in life-style and nutritional requirements among the age categories. But with simple adjustments, any menu here can serve a family containing people of all ages. Adults and older adults can follow any menu as long as they stay at the right calorie level; adolescents must add a few portions to any adult or older-adult menu in order to meet their Setpoint requirements.

The recipes are for 81 items included on these menus. Their taste-temptingness underscores the pleasant fact that eating to lose weight can be enjoyable.

## Setpoint Guide to Ingredients

| Ingredient | Amount | Setpoint Portion |
|---|---|---|
| Butter/Margarine | ½ cup (one stick) | 12 A Bonus |
| | 2 tbsp | 3 A Bonus |
| Vegetable Oil/Shortening | ½ cup | 14 A Bonus |
| | 2 tbsp | 3 A Bonus |
| Mayonnaise | ½ cup | 12 A Bonus |
| Mayonnaise, imitation | ½ cup | 4 A Bonus |
| Cream Cheese | 8 oz pkg | 12 A Bonus |
| | 3 oz pkg | 4½ A Bonus |
| | 1 tbsp | 1 A Bonus |
| Sour Cream | 1 cup | 8 A Bonus |
| Yogurt, plain, low-fat or whole | 1 cup | 1 Milk/Dairy Products + ½ A Bonus |
| Half-and-Half | 1 cup | 5 A Bonus |
| Cream, light | 1 cup | 7 A Bonus |
| Cream, heavy | 1 cup | 12 A Bonus |
| Sweetened Condensed Milk | 1 cup | 3 Milk/Dairy Products + 10 A Bonus |
| Evaporated Whole Milk, canned (not reconstituted) | ½ cup | 1 Milk/Dairy Products + 1 A Bonus |
| Egg, large | 1 | ½ Meat/Fish/Poultry |
| Sugar, white or brown | ½ cup | 6 A Bonus |
| Sugar, confectioners (unsifted) | 1 cup | 7 A Bonus |
| Honey | ¼ cup | 4 A Bonus |
| Syrup, maple | ½ cup | 6 A Bonus |
| Syrup, corn | ½ cup | 7 A Bonus |
| Flour, enriched (unsifted) | 1 cup | 7 Bread/Cereals/Starchy Foods |
| | 1 tbsp | ½ Bread/Cereals/Starchy Foods |

| Ingredient | Amount | Setpoint Portion |
|---|---|---|
| Oats, dry | 1 cup | 4½ Bread/Cereals/Starchy Foods |
| Cornmeal/Grits, dry | 1 cup | 8 Bread/Cereals/Starchy Foods |
| Bread Crumbs, dry | ½ cup | 3 Bread/Cereals/Starchy Foods |
| Graham Cracker Crumbs, dry | ½ cup | 3 Bread/Cereals/Starchy Foods |
| Nuts, chopped (Walnuts, Peanuts, Almonds, Pecans) | ½ cup | 6 A Bonus |
| Coconut, unsweetened, dried, flaked, or shredded | 1 cup | 9 A Bonus |
| Chocolate, baking, unsweetened | 1 oz square 1 cup grated | 2 A Bonus 10 A Bonus |
| Chocolate Chips, semisweet | 1 cup or 6 oz pkg | 13 A Bonus |
| Marshmallows, miniature | 1 cup | 2 A Bonus |
| Raisins, packed | ½ cup | 6 Fruits |
| Tapioca | 2 tbsp | 1 A Bonus |

## Measurement Conversion Table

1 tbsp = 3 tsp
2 tbsp = 1 fl oz
⅓ cup = 5 tbsp + 1 tsp
¾ cup = 12 tbsp
1 cup = 16 tbsp = ½ pt = 8 fl oz
2 cups = 1 pt = 16 fl oz
1 quart = 2 pt = 4 cups
4 quarts = 1 gal
1 oz = 28 grams
1 pound = 16 oz

# Setpoint Menus—Specially for Adults

## ADULTS

### Day One—Monday

| | 1200 Calories | 1500 Calories | 1800 Calories | 2100 Calories | 2400 Calories |
|---|---|---|---|---|---|
| **Breakfast** | | | | | |
| Orange-flavored breakfast beverage | 6 fl oz | 6 fl oz | 6 fl oz | 6 fl oz | 6 fl oz |
| Whole wheat and bran cereal with apples and cinnamon | ½ cup | ½ cup | 1 cup | 1 cup | 1 cup |
| Milk | Skim or 1% lowfat, 1 cup | Skim or 1% lowfat, 1 cup | Skim or 1% lowfat, 1 cup | 2% lowfat, 1 cup | 2% lowfat, 1 cup |
| Cinnamon bread toast | 1 slice | 1 slice | 2 slices | 2 slices | 2 slices |
| Butter | None | 1 tsp | 2 tsp | 2 tsp | 2 tsp |
| Coffee, regular or decaffeinated | * | * | * | * | * |
| **Lunch** | | | | | |
| Sliced turkey sandwich | | | | | |
| Sliced turkey breast | 3 oz | 3 oz | 3 oz | 3 oz | 3 oz |
| Bread | 2 slices | 2 slices | 2 slices | 2 slices | 2 slices |
| Lettuce | * | * | * | * | * |
| Mayonnaise | 2 tsp | 2 tsp | 2 tsp | 2 tsp | 2 tsp |
| Tossed salad | 1½ cups | 1½ cups | 1½ cups | 1½ cups | 1½ cups |
| Salad dressing | Low-calorie, 1 tbsp | Regular, 1 tbsp | Regular, 1 tbsp | Regular, 1 tbsp | Regular, 1 tbsp |

| | | | | | |
|---|---|---|---|---|---|
| Cantaloupe with ice cream | ¼ melon | ½ melon | ½ melon | ½ melon | ½ melon |
| | None | None | None | ½ cup | ½ cup |
| Coffee, regular or decaffeinated | * | * | * | * | * |
| *Dinner* | | | | | |
| Tomato bouillon | | | | | |
| Tomato juice | ¼ cup | ¼ cup | ¼ cup | ¼ cup | ¼ cup |
| Bouillon | ¼ cup | ¼ cup | ¼ cup | ¼ cup | ¼ cup |
| •Pork Chops w/Corn and Zucchini | 1 serving | 1 serving | 1 serving | 1 serving | 1 serving |
| Spinach salad w/ onion rings | 1½ cups | 1½ cups | 1½ cups | 1½ cups | 1½ cups |
| Salad dressing | Low-calorie, 1 tbsp | Low-calorie, 1 tbsp | Regular, 1 tbsp | Regular, 1 tbsp | Regular, 1 tbsp |
| Baked apple (with lemon and dash of cinnamon) | 1 small | None | None | None | None |
| Apple pie | None | 1/12 pie | 1/12 pie | 1/12 pie | 1/6 pie |
| Coffee, regular or decaffeinated | * | * | * | * | * |
| *Snacks* | | | | | |
| Fruit shake | Skim or 1% lowfat, 1 cup | Skim or 1% lowfat, 1 cup | Skim or 1% lowfat, 1 cup | 2% lowfat, 1 cup | 2% lowfat, 1 cup |
| Milk | | | | | |
| Strawberries or Banana | ¾ cup or ½ small | ¾ cup or ½ small | ¾ cup or ½ small | ¾ cup or ½ small | ¾ cup or ½ small |
| Cola | None | None | None | 6 fl oz | 12 fl oz |

*As desired
•Recipe on page 246

## Day Two—Tuesday

### ADULTS

| | 1200 Calories | 1500 Calories | 1800 Calories | 2100 Calories | 2400 Calories |
|---|---|---|---|---|---|
| *Breakfast* | | | | | |
| Cranberry-apple juice | ⅔ cup | ⅔ cup | ⅔ cup | ⅔ cup | ⅔ cup |
| Toasted English muffin | 1 whole | 1 whole | 1 whole | 1 whole | 1 whole |
| Swiss cheese, melted | ½ oz | 1 oz | 1 oz | 1 oz | 1 oz |
| Bacon | None | None | None | None | 1 strip |
| Milk | Skim or 1% lowfat, 1 cup | Skim or 1% lowfat, 1 cup | Skim or 1% lowfat, 1 cup | 2% lowfat, 1 cup | 2% lowfat, 1 cup |
| Coffee, regular or decaffeinated | * | * | * | * | * |
| *Lunch* | | | | | |
| Hamburger on roll | 2 oz (small) | | | | |
| Lean hamburger | | 3 oz | 3 oz | 4 oz | 4 oz |
| Hamburger roll | 1 | 1 | 1 | 1 | 1 |
| Tomato slices | 2 | 2 | 2 | 2 | 2 |
| Lettuce, onion slice | * | * | * | * | * |
| Mustard, catsup | 1 tbsp | 1 tbsp | 1 tbsp | 1 tbsp | 1 tbsp |
| French fries | None | None | 10 medium | 10 medium | 10 medium |
| Carrot/cabbage slaw | ¾ cup | ¾ cup | ¾ cup | ¾ cup | ¾ cup |
| Vinegar | * | * | * | * | * |
| Mayonnaise | None | 1 tbsp | 1 tbsp | 1 tbsp | 1 tbsp |
| Blueberries | ½ cup | ½ cup | ½ cup | None | None |

| | None | None | None | 1/12 pie | ⅙ pie |
|---|---|---|---|---|---|
| Coconut custard pie | None | None | None | 1/12 pie | ⅙ pie |
| Coffee, regular or decaffeinated | * | * | * | * | * |
| **Dinner** | | | | | |
| •Turkey Divan | 1 serving | 1 serving | 1 serving | 1 serving | 1 serving |
| Hearts of romaine salad | 1½ cups | 1½ cups | 1½ cups | 1½ cups | 1½ cups |
| Salad dressing | Low-calorie, 1 tbsp | Low-calorie, 1 tbsp | Regular, 1 tbsp | Regular, 1 tbsp | Regular, 1 tbsp |
| Citrus fruit sections | ½ cup | ½ cup | ½ cup | ½ cup | ½ cup |
| Fruit flavor gelatin cubes | ¼ cup | ¼ cup | ¼ cup | ¼ cup | ¼ cup |
| Dinner roll | None | 1 small | 1 small | 1 small | 1 small |
| Butter | None | 1 tsp | 1 tsp | 1 tsp | 1 tsp |
| Coffee, regular or decaffeinated | * | * | * | * | * |
| **Snacks** | | | | | |
| Ice milk sprinkled with | ½ cup | ½ cup | ½ cup | ½ cup | ½ cup |
| crunchy nutlike cereal nuggets | 2 tbsp | 2 tbsp | 2 tbsp | 2 tbsp | 2 tbsp |
| Blueberries | None | None | None | ½ cup | ½ cup |
| Frozen whipped topping | None | None | None | None | 2 tbsp |

*As desired
•Recipe on page 251

**ADULTS**

## Day Three—Wednesday

| | 1200 Calories | 1500 Calories | 1800 Calories | 2100 Calories | 2400 Calories |
|---|---|---|---|---|---|
| **Breakfast** | | | | | |
| Orange | 1 small | 1 small | 1 small | 1 small | 1 large |
| Poached egg | 1 | 1 | 1 | 1 | 1 |
| Whole wheat toast | 2 slices | 2 slices | 2 slices | 2 slices | 2 slices |
| Butter | None | 1 tsp | 1 tsp | 1 tsp | 1 tsp |
| Milk | Skim or 1% lowfat, 1 cup | Skim or 1% lowfat, 1 cup | Skim or 1% lowfat, 1 cup | 2% lowfat, 1 cup | 2% lowfat, 1 cup |
| Coffee, regular or decaffeinated | * | * | * | * | * |
| **Lunch** | | | | | |
| Sausage pizza | ⅙ large pie | ⅙ large pie | ⅙ large pie | ⅓ large pie | ⅓ large pie |
| Tossed salad | ¾ cup | ¾ cup | ¾ cup | ¾ cup | ¾ cup |
| Salad dressing | Low-calorie, 1 tbsp | Low-calorie, 1 tbsp | Regular, 1 tbsp | Regular, 1 tbsp | Regular, 1 tbsp |
| Fruit cup | ½ cup | ½ cup | ½ cup | ½ cup | ½ cup |
| Coffee, regular or decaffeinated | * | * | * | * | * |
| **Dinner** | | | | | |
| •Fettuccine Carbonara | 1 serving | 1½ servings | 1½ servings | 1½ servings | 1½ servings |
| Salad greens with radishes and onions | 1 cup | 1 cup | 1 cup | 1 cup | 1 cup |
| Salad dressing | Low-calorie, 1 tbsp | Regular, 1 tbsp | Regular, 1 tbsp | Regular, 1 tbsp | Regular, 1 tbsp |
| Nectarine | 1 small | 1 small | 1 medium | 1 medium | 1 medium |
| Coffee, regular or decaffeinated | * | * | * | * | * |

| Snacks | | | | | |
|---|---|---|---|---|---|
| Carrot and celery sticks | ½ cup | ½ cup | ½ cup | ½ cup | ½ cup |
| Dry white wine | 3 fl oz | 3 fl oz | 3 fl oz | 3 fl oz | 3 fl oz |
| Frosted cupcake | None | None | None | None | 1 |
| Ginger ale | None | None | 6 fl oz | 6 fl oz | 12 fl oz |

*As desired
•Recipe on page 234

**ADULTS**

## Day Four—Thursday

| | 1200 Calories | 1500 Calories | 1800 Calories | 2100 Calories | 2400 Calories |
|---|---|---|---|---|---|
| *Breakfast* | | | | | |
| Grapefruit juice | ½ cup | ½ cup | ½ cup | ½ cup | ½ cup |
| Toasted bagel | 1 whole | 1 whole | 1 whole | 1 whole | 1 whole |
| Cream cheese *or* | 1 tbsp *or* | 2 tbsp *or* | 2 tbsp *or* | 2 tbsp *or* | 2 tbsp *or* |
| Brie | 2 tbsp | 4 tbsp | 4 tbsp | 4 tbsp | 4 tbsp |
| Milk | Skim or 1% lowfat, 1 cup | Skim or 1% lowfat, 1 cup | Skim or 1% lowfat, 1 cup | 2% lowfat, 1 cup | 2% lowfat, 1 cup |
| | | | | | |
| Coffee, regular or decaffeinated | * | * | * | * | * |
| *Lunch* | | | | | |
| Bacon, lettuce, and tomato sandwich | | | | | |
| Bacon | 4 strips | 4 strips | 4 strips | 4 strips | 4 strips |
| Lettuce | * | * | * | * | * |
| Tomato | 3 slices | 3 slices | 3 slices | 3 slices | 3 slices |
| Mayonnaise | 2 tsp | 2 tsp | 2 tsp | 2 tsp | 1 tbsp |
| Toast | 2 slices | 2 slices | 2 slices | 2 slices | 2 slices |
| Celery sticks | ½ cup | ½ cup | ½ cup | ½ cup | ½ cup |
| Strawberries | ¾ cup | ¾ cup | ¾ cup | ¾ cup | ¾ cup |
| Pound cake | None | None | None | ¾-inch slice | ¾-inch slice |
| Frozen whipped topping | None | None | None | 3 tbsp | 3 tbsp |
| Coffee, regular or decaffeinated | * | * | * | * | * |

| | | | | | |
|---|---|---|---|---|---|
| **Dinner** | | | | | |
| •Mexican Beef Kebabs | 1 serving | 1 serving | 1 serving | 1 serving | 1 serving |
| Marinated artichoke hearts | ¼ cup | ½ cup | ½ cup | ½ cup | ½ cup |
| Salad dressing | Low-calorie, 1 tbsp | Regular, 1 tbsp | Regular, 1 tbsp | Regular, 1 tbsp | Regular, 1 tbsp |
| Corn muffin | None | 1 | 1 | 1 | 1 |
| Pineapple chunks topped with | ½ cup | ¾ cup | ¾ cup | ¾ cup | ¾ cup |
| hearty granola cereal | None | None | ⅓ cup | ⅓ cup | ⅓ cup |
| Coffee, regular or decaffeinated | * | * | * | * | * |
| **Snacks** | | | | | |
| Milk | Skim or 1% lowfat, 1 cup | Skim or 1% lowfat, 1 cup | Skim or 1% lowfat, 1 cup | 2% lowfat, 1 cup | 2% lowfat, 1 cup |
| Cookie | 1 medium | 1 medium | 2 medium | 2 medium | 3 medium |
| Ice cream | None | None | None | None | ¾ cup |
| Wafer cone | None | None | None | None | 1 |

*As desired
•Recipe on page 242

## Day Five—Friday

**ADULTS**

| | 1200 Calories | 1500 Calories | 1800 Calories | 2100 Calories | 2400 Calories |
|---|---|---|---|---|---|
| *Breakfast* | | | | | |
| Banana *or* | ½ small *or* | ½ small *or* | ½ small *or* | 1 small *or* | 1 small *or* |
| blueberries | ½ cup | ½ cup | ½ cup | 1 cup | 1 cup |
| Crunchy nutlike cereal nuggets | ¼ cup | ¼ cup | ¼ cup | ¼ cup | ¼ cup |
| Yogurt | Plain lowfat, 1 cup | Vanilla yogurt, 1 cup | Vanilla yogurt, 1 cup | Vanilla yogurt, 1 cup | Vanilla yogurt, 1 cup |
| Coffee, regular or decaffeinated | * | * | * | * | * |
| *Lunch* | | | | | |
| Chef's salad | | | | | |
| Chicken *or* turkey breast | 1½ oz | 1½ oz | 1½ oz | 1½ oz | 1½ oz |
| Smoked cooked ham | 1 oz | 1 oz | 1 oz | 1½ oz | 1½ oz |
| Swiss cheese | 1 oz | 1 oz | 1 oz | 1½ oz | 1½ oz |
| Lettuce | 1½ cups | 1½ cups | 1½ cups | 1½ cups | 1½ cups |
| Tomatoes and onion | ⅓ cup | ⅓ cup | ⅓ cup | ⅓ cup | ⅓ cup |
| Salad dressing | Low-calorie, 2 tbsp | Regular, 2 tbsp | Regular, 2 tbsp | Regular, 2 tbsp | Regular, 2 tbsp |
| Italian bread | 1 slice | 1 slice | 1 slice | 2 slices | 2 slices |
| Orange sections | ½ cup | ½ cup | ½ cup | ½ cup | ½ cup |
| Coffee, regular or decaffeinated | * | * | * | * | * |

| | | | | | |
|---|---|---|---|---|---|
| *Dinner* | | | | | |
| Tomato juice | ½ cup | ½ cup | ½ cup | ¾ cup | ¾ cup |
| Poached haddock fillet | 4 oz | 4 oz | 4 oz | 4 oz | 4 oz |
| Almonds | None | None | None | 5 | 5 |
| •Savory Lemon Rice | ⅔ cup | ⅔ cup | ⅔ cup | ⅔ cup | ⅔ cup |
| Spinach | ½ cup | ½ cup | ½ cup | ¾ cup | ¾ cup |
| Sliced cucumber with dill | ½ cup | ½ cup | ½ cup | ½ cup | ½ cup |
| Wine vinegar | None | * | None | None | None |
| Mayonnaise | None | None | 2 tsp | 2 tsp | 2 tsp |
| French bread | None | 1 slice | 1 slice | 1 slice | 1 slice |
| Butter | None | None | None | None | 1 tsp |
| Chocolate Flavor Pudding | ½ cup | ½ cup | ½ cup | ½ cup | ½ cup |
| Tart shell | None | None | 1 | 1 | 1 |
| Walnuts | None | None | None | 2 | 2 |
| Frozen whipped topping | None | None | None | None | 3 tbsp |
| Coffee, regular or decaffeinated | * | * | * | * | * |
| *Snacks* | | | | | |
| Pear | ½ medium | ½ medium | ½ medium | ½ medium | ½ medium |
| Fruit flavor sugar-free soft drink mix made with club soda, if desired | 8 fl oz | 8 fl oz | 8 fl oz | 8 fl oz | 8 fl oz |
| Lemon-lime soda | None | None | None | None | 12 fl oz |

*As desired
•Recipe on page 262

**ADULTS**

## Day Six—Saturday

| | 1200 Calories | 1500 Calories | 1800 Calories | 2100 Calories | 2400 Calories |
|---|---|---|---|---|---|
| *Breakfast* | | | | | |
| Pineapple juice | ⅔ cup | ⅔ cup | ⅔ cup | ⅔ cup | ⅔ cup |
| Pancakes | 2 medium | 4 medium | 4 medium | 4 medium | 4 medium |
| Waffle syrup | 1 tbsp | 2 tbsp | 2 tbsp | 2 tbsp | 2 tbsp |
| Butter | None | 2 tsp | 2 tsp | 2 tsp | 2 tbsp |
| Breakfast sausage links | None | None | None | None | 4 links |
| Milk | Skim or 1% lowfat, 1 cup | Skim or 1% lowfat, 1 cup | Skim or 1% lowfat, 1 cup | 2% lowfat, 1 cup | 2% lowfat, 1 cup |
| Coffee, regular or decaffeinated | * | * | * | * | * |
| *Lunch* | | | | | |
| Beef taco | | | | | |
| Taco shell | 1 | 1 | 1 | 2 | 2 |
| Ground beef, lean | 1½ oz | 1½ oz | 1½ oz | 1½ oz each | 1½ oz each |
| Tomato, chopped | * | * | * | * | * |
| Lettuce, shredded | * | * | * | * | * |
| Monterey cheese, grated | ¾ oz | ¾ oz | ¾ oz | ¾ oz each | ¾ oz each |
| Taco sauce | * | * | * | * | * |
| Carrot sticks | ½ cup | ½ cup | ½ cup | ½ cup | ½ cup |
| Apple | 1 small | 1 small | 1 large | 1 large | 1 large |
| Coffee, regular or decaffeinated | * | * | * | * | * |
| *Dinner* | | | | | |
| Consommé | 1 cup | 1 cup | 1 cup | 1 cup | 1 cup |
| Broiled chicken breast | 3 oz | 4½ oz | 4½ oz | 6 oz | 6 oz |

| | | | | |
|---|---|---|---|---|
| Stuffing with mushrooms | ½ cup | ½ cup | ¾ cup | ¾ cup | ¾ cup |
| Deluxe baby broccoli spears | ½ cup | ½ cup | ½ cup | ½ cup | ½ cup |
| Breadsticks | 1 medium | 2 medium | 2 medium | 2 medium | 2 medium |
| •Creamy Coffee Delight | ½ cup | ½ cup | ½ cup | ½ cup | ½ cup |
| Coffee, regular or decaffeinated | * | * | * | * | * |
| *Snacks* | | | | | |
| Celery and green pepper strips | ½ cup | ½ cup | ½ cup | ½ cup | ½ cup |
| Dip made with | None | None | ½ cup | ½ cup | ½ cup |
| 1% lowfat cottage cheese and | | | | | |
| parsley | | | | | |
| Club soda with lime juice | 8 fl oz | 8 fl oz | 8 fl oz | 8 fl oz | 8 fl oz |
| Lemonade flavor drink | None | None | 6 fl oz | 6 fl oz | 12 fl oz |

*As desired
•Recipe on page 270

## Day Seven—Sunday

ADULTS

| | 1200 Calories | 1500 Calories | 1800 Calories | 2100 Calories | 2400 Calories |
|---|---|---|---|---|---|
| *"Eye Opener" Breakfast* | | | | | |
| Orange juice | ⅓ cup | ⅔ cup | ⅔ cup | ⅔ cup | ⅔ cup |
| Croissant | 1 small or ½ medium | 1 medium | 1 medium | 1 medium | 1 medium |
| Jam | None | None | 1 tsp | 2 tsp | 2 tsp |
| Coffee, regular or decaffeinated | * | * | * | * | * |
| *Brunch* | | | | | |
| Quiche | ⅙ pie | ⅙ pie | ⅙ pie | ⅙ pie | ⅓ pie |
| Watercress, lettuce, endive salad | 2 cups | 2 cups | 2 cups | 2 cups | 2 cups |
| Salad dressing | Low-calorie, 1 tbsp | Regular, 2 tsp | Regular, 1 tbsp | Regular, 1 tbsp | Regular, 1 tbsp |
| Cherry flavor gelatin with Bing cherries | ½ cup 10 | ½ cup 10 | ½ cup 10 | ½ cup 10 | ½ cup 10 |
| and brandy | ½ tsp | ½ tsp | ½ tsp | ½ tsp | ½ tsp |
| Cream | None | None | 1 tbsp | 1 tbsp | 1 tbsp |
| Coffee, regular or decaffeinated | * | * | * | * | * |
| *Dinner* | | | | | |
| •Ginger Beef with Stir-Fry Vegetables | 1 serving | 1 serving | 1½ servings | 1½ servings | 1½ servings |
| Rice | ⅔ cup | ⅔ cup | ⅔ cup | 1 cup | 1 cup |
| Tomato and green onion salad | ½ cup | ½ cup | 1 cup | 1 cup | 1 cup |
| Salad dressing | Low-calorie, 1 tbsp | Regular, 2 tsp | Regular, 1 tbsp | Regular, 1 tbsp | Regular, 1 tbsp |

| | | | | | |
|---|---|---|---|---|---|
| Diced apples, seedless grapes, mandarin oranges, and bananas | ½ cup | ½ cup | ½ cup | 1 cup | 1 cup |
| Coffee, regular or decaffeinated | * | * | * | * | * |
| *"Lite" Supper* | | | | | |
| Pita pocket sandwich | | | | | |
| Pita bread | 1 small | 1 small | 1 small | 1 large | 1 large |
| Sliced chicken breast | 1½ oz | 1½ oz | 1½ oz | 3 oz | 3 oz |
| Mayonnaise | Low-calorie, 1 tsp | Regular, 2 tsp | Regular, 2 tsp | Regular, 1 tbsp | Regular, 1 tbsp |
| Lettuce | * | * | * | * | * |
| Milk | Skim or 1% lowfat, 1 cup | Skim or 1% lowfat, 1 cup | Skim or 1% lowfat, 1 cup | 2% lowfat, 1 cup | 2% lowfat, 1 cup |
| *Snacks* | | | | | |
| Carrot sticks | 2 | 2 | 2 | 2 | 2 |
| Dry wine | 3 fl oz | 3 fl oz | 3 fl oz | 3 fl oz | 4 fl oz |

*As desired
•Recipe on page 237

## Day Eight—Monday

**ADULTS**

| | 1200 Calories | 1500 Calories | 1800 Calories | 2100 Calories | 2400 Calories |
|---|---|---|---|---|---|
| *Breakfast* | | | | | |
| Orange flavor breakfast beverage | 6 fl oz | 6 fl oz | 6 fl oz | 6 fl oz | 6 fl oz |
| Crisp whole wheat flakes | ¾ cup | ¾ cup | ¾ cup | ¾ cup | ¾ cup |
| Milk | Skim or 1% lowfat, 1 cup | Skim or 1% lowfat, 1 cup | Skim or 1% lowfat, 1 cup | 2% lowfat, 1 cup | 2% lowfat, 1 cup |
| Plain Danish pastry | None | None | ⅛ ring | ⅛ ring | ⅛ ring |
| Coffee, regular or decaffeinated | * | * | * | * | * |
| *Lunch* | | | | | |
| Cocktail vegetable juice | ½ cup | ½ cup | ½ cup | ½ cup | ½ cup |
| Roast beef sandwich | | | | | |
| Lean roast beef | 2 oz | 3 oz | 3 oz | 4 oz | 4 oz |
| Rye bread | 2 slices | 2 slices | 2 slices | 2 slices | 2 slices |
| Lettuce, mustard | * | * | * | * | * |
| Mayonnaise | None | 2 tsp | 2 tsp | 1 tbsp | 1 tbsp |
| Cole slaw | None | ½ cup | ½ cup | ½ cup | ¾ cup |
| Melon wedge with lemon | ¼ small | ¼ small | ¼ small | ¼ small | ½ small |
| Coffee, regular or decaffeinated | * | * | * | * | * |
| *Dinner* | | | | | |
| •Pasta Primavera | 1 serving | 1 serving | 1 serving | 1 serving | 1 serving |
| Sliced cooked ham | 1 oz | 1½ oz | 1½ oz | 1½ oz | 1½ oz |
| Sliced turkey breast | 1½ oz | 1½ oz | 1½ oz | 1½ oz | 1½ oz |
| Tomato wedges on lettuce | ½ cup | ½ cup | ½ cup | ½ cup | ½ cup |

|  |  |  |  |  |  |
|---|---|---|---|---|---|
| Italian bread | None | None | 1 slice | 1 slice | 1 slice |
| Blueberries | 1/2 cup | 1/2 cup | 1/2 cup | 1/2 cup | 1/2 cup |
| Angel food cake | None | None | None | 1/8 cake | 1/8 cake |
| Coffee, regular or decaffeinated | * | * | * | * | * |
| *Snacks* |  |  |  |  |  |
| Whipped fruit-flavor gelatin with sliced banana | 3/4 cup 1/2 small | 3/4 cup 1/2 small | 3/4 cup 1/2 small | 3/4 cup 1/2 small | 3/4 cup 1/2 small |
| English muffin | None | 1/2 muffin | 1/2 muffin | 1/2 muffin | 1/2 muffin |
| Butter | None | 1 tsp | 1 tsp | 1 tsp | 1 tsp |
| Cola | None | None | None | None | 12 fl oz |
| Milk | Skim or 1% lowfat, 1/2 cup | Skim or 1% lowfat, 1/2 cup | Skim or 1% lowfat, 1/2 cup | 2% lowfat, 1/2 cup | 2% lowfat, 1/2 cup |

*As desired
•Recipe on page 245

**ADULTS**

## Day Nine—Tuesday

| | 1200 Calories | 1500 Calories | 1800 Calories | 2100 Calories | 2400 Calories |
|---|---|---|---|---|---|
| *Breakfast* | | | | | |
| Banana | ½ small | ½ small | 1 small | 1 medium | 1 medium |
| Bran flakes with raisins | ½ cup | 1 cup | 1 cup | 1½ cups | 1½ cups |
| Milk | Skim or 1% lowfat, 1 cup | Skim or 1% lowfat, 1 cup | Skim or 1% lowfat, 1 cup | 2% lowfat, 1 cup | 2% lowfat, 1 cup |
| Coffee, regular or decaffeinated | * | * | * | * | * |
| *Lunch* | | | | | |
| Bologna sandwich on pumpernickel | | | | | |
| Bologna | 2 slices | 2 slices | 2 slices | 2 slices | 3 slices |
| Pumpernickel bread | 2 slices | 2 slices | 2 slices | 2 slices | 2 slices |
| Mustard | * | * | * | * | * |
| Sauerkraut | ½ cup | ½ cup | ½ cup | ½ cup | ½ cup |
| Bread and butter pickle chips | 4 chips | 4 chips | 4 chips | 4 chips | 4 chips |
| Potato chips | None | None | None | None | 15 chips |
| Orange | 1 small | 1 small | 1 large | 1 large | 1 large |
| Lemonade flavor drink | None | None | 12 fl oz | 12 fl oz | 12 fl oz |
| Coffee, regular or decaffeinated | * | * | * | * | * |
| *Dinner* | | | | | |
| Baked lemon flounder | 4 oz | 6 oz | 6 oz | 6 oz | 6 oz |
| Butter | 2 tsp | 2 tsp | 2 tsp | 2 tsp | 2 tsp |
| Green peas | ½ cup | ½ cup | ½ cup | ¾ cup | ¾ cup |
| Broiled tomato | 1 small | 1 small | 1 small | 1 small | 1 small |

| | | | | | |
|---|---|---|---|---|---|
| Mixed green salad | 2 cups | 2 cups | 2 cups | 2 cups | 2 cups |
| Salad dressing | Low-calorie, 1 tbsp | Regular, 1 tbsp | Regular, 1 tbsp | Regular, 1 tbsp | Regular, 1 tbsp |
| •Carrot Pudding Cake with Orange Cream Cheese Frosting | ½ in. slice | ½ in. slice | ½ in. slice | ½ in. slice | ½ in. slice |
| Coffee, regular or decaffeinated | * | * | * | * | * |
| *Snacks* | | | | | |
| Milk | Skim or 1% lowfat, 1 cup | Skim or 1% lowfat, 1 cup | Skim or 1% lowfat, 1 cup | 2% lowfat, 1 cup | 2% lowfat, 1 cup |
| Peach | 1 medium | 1 medium | 1 large | 1 large | 1 large |
| Graham crackers | None | 3 squares | 4 squares | 4 squares | 5 squares |
| Peanuts | None | None | None | 20 large | 20 large |

*As desired

•Recipe on page 267

## ADULTS

### Day Ten—Wednesday

| | 1200 Calories | 1500 Calories | 1800 Calories | 2100 Calories | 2400 Calories |
|---|---|---|---|---|---|
| **Breakfast** | | | | | |
| Apple juice | ⅓ cup | ⅓ cup | ⅔ cup | 1 cup | 1 cup |
| Whole wheat toast | 1 slice | 1 slice | 1 slice | 1 slice | 1 slice |
| Gouda cheese | 1½ oz | 1½ oz | 1½ oz | 1½ oz | 1½ oz |
| Omelet | None | None | 1 | 1 | 1 |
| Egg | None | None | | | |
| Butter | None | None | 1 tsp | 1 tsp | 1 tsp |
| Milk | Skim or 1% lowfat, 1 cup | Skim or 1% lowfat, 1 cup | Skim or 1% lowfat, 1 cup | 2% lowfat, 1 cup | 2% lowfat, 1 cup |
| Coffee, regular or decaffeinated | * | * | * | * | * |
| **Lunch** | | | | | |
| Chili with beans | 1 cup | 1 cup | 1 cup | 1½ cups | 1½ cups |
| Saltines | None | 3 | 3 | 6 | 6 |
| Tossed vegetable salad | 1½ cups | 1½ cups | 1½ cups | 1½ cups | 1½ cups |
| Salad dressing | Low-calorie, 1 tbsp | Regular, 1 tbsp | Regular, 1 tbsp | Regular, 1 tbsp | Regular, 1 tbsp |
| Fruit cup | ½ cup | ½ cup | ½ cup | ½ cup | ½ cup |
| Sherbet | None | None | ½ cup | ½ cup | ½ cup |
| Coffee, regular or decaffeinated | * | * | * | * | * |
| **Dinner** | | | | | |
| •Superb Pepper Steak | 1 serving | 1 serving | 1 serving | 1 serving | 1 serving |
| Farm fresh vegetables | ½ cup | ½ cup | ½ cup | ½ cup | ½ cup |

| | | | | | |
|---|---|---|---|---|---|
| Spinach salad with sliced mushrooms | 1 cup | 1 cup | 1 cup | 1 cup | 1 cup |
| Salad dressing | Low-calorie, 1 tbsp | Regular, 1 tbsp | Regular, 1 tbsp | Regular, 1 tbsp | Regular, 1 tbsp |
| Dinner roll | None | 1 small | 1 small | 1 small | 1 small |
| Butter | None | None | None | 1 tsp | 1 tsp |
| Apricot halves | 4 halves | 4 halves | 4 halves | 8 halves | 8 halves |
| Coffee, regular or decaffeinated | * | * | * | * | * |
| *Snacks* | | | | | |
| Zucchini strips | ½ cup | ½ cup | ½ cup | ½ cup | ½ cup |
| Wine *or* | 3 fl oz *or* | 4½ fl oz *or* | 4½ fl oz *or* | 4½ fl oz *or* | 4½ fl oz *or* |
| Light beer | 8 fl oz | 12 fl oz | 12 fl oz | 12 fl oz | 12 fl oz |
| Dip made from sour cream with chives | None | None | None | None | ¼ cup |
| Candy bar | None | None | None | None | 1½ oz bar |

* As desired
• Recipe on page 248

## Day Eleven—Thursday

**ADULTS**

| | 1200 Calories | 1500 Calories | 1800 Calories | 2100 Calories | 2400 Calories |
|---|---|---|---|---|---|
| *Breakfast* | | | | | |
| Orange | 1 small | 1 small | 1 large | 1 large | 1 large |
| Raisin bread toast | 2 slices | 2 slices | 2 slices | 2 slices | 2 slices |
| Cream cheese | 2 tbsp | 2 tbsp | 2 tbsp | 2 tbsp | 2 tbsp |
| Milk | Skim or 1% lowfat, 1 cup | Skim or 1% lowfat, 1 cup | Skim or 1% lowfat, 1 cup | 2% lowfat, 1 cup | 2% lowfat, 1 cup |
| Coffee, regular or decaffeinated | * | * | * | * | * |
| *Lunch* | | | | | |
| Frankfurter with bun *or* | 1 medium | 1 medium | 1 medium | 1 medium | 1 medium |
| Baked beans | 1 *or* | 1 *or* | 1 *and* | 1 *and* | 1 *and* |
| Beef frank or wiener | ½ cup | ½ cup | ¼ cup | ½ cup | ½ cup |
| Hot dog bun *or* | 2 tsp | 2 tsp | 2 tsp | 2 tsp | 2 tsp |
| Baked beans | ½ cup | ½ cup | ½ cup | ½ cup | ½ cup |
| Mustard, sweet relish | | | | | |
| Sauerkraut | 1 small | 1 medium | 1 medium | 1 large | 1 large |
| Apple | | | | | |
| Milk | Skim or 1% lowfat, 1 cup | Skim or 1% lowfat, 1 cup | Skim or 1% lowfat, 1 cup | 2% lowfat, 1 cup | 2% lowfat, 1 cup |
| Coffee, regular or decaffeinated | * | * | * | * | * |

| | 1 serving | 1 serving | 1 serving | 1½ servings | 1½ servings |
|---|---|---|---|---|---|
| **Dinner** | | | | | |
| •Chicken Ratatouille | 1 serving | 1 serving | 1 serving | 1½ servings | 1½ servings |
| Watercress and shredded carrot salad | 1 cup | 1 cup | 1 cup | 1 cup | 1 cup |
| with Feta cheese | None | None | ½ oz | ½ oz | ½ oz |
| Salad dressing | Low-calorie, 1 tbsp | Low-calorie, 1 tbsp | Regular, 1 tbsp | Regular, 1 tbsp | Regular, 1 tbsp |
| Hard roll | None | 1 small | 1 small | 1 small | 2 small |
| Butter | None | 1 tsp | 1 tsp | 1 tsp | 2 tsp |
| Seedless grapes and banana with orange juice | ½ cup | ½ cup | ½ cup | 1 cup | 1 cup |
| Coffee, regular or decaffeinated | * | * | * | * | * |
| **Snack** | | | | | |
| Roman style instant coffee beverage | 6 fl oz | 6 fl oz | 6 fl oz | 6 fl oz | 6 fl oz |
| Brownie | None | 1 medium | 1 medium | 1 medium | 2 medium |
| Fruit flavor sugar-sweetened soft drink | None | None | None | None | 6 fl oz |

*As desired
•Recipe on page 224

**ADULTS**

## Day Twelve—Friday

| | *1200 Calories* | *1500 Calories* | *1800 Calories* | *2100 Calories* | *2400 Calories* |
|---|---|---|---|---|---|
| *Breakfast* | | | | | |
| Apricot nectar | ⅓ cup | ⅓ cup | ⅔ cup | ⅔ cup | ⅔ cup |
| Oatmeal with cinnamon | ¾ cup | ¾ cup | ¾ cup | ¾ cup | ¾ cup |
| Brown sugar | None | 2 tsp | 2 tsp | 2 tsp | 2 tsp |
| Doughnut holes | None | 3 | 3 | 3 | 3 |
| Milk | Skim or 1% lowfat, 1 cup | Skim or 1% lowfat, 1 cup | Skim or 1% lowfat, 1 cup | 2% lowfat, 1 cup | 2% lowfat, 1 cup |
| Coffee, regular or decaffeinated | * | * | * | * | * |
| *Lunch* | | | | | |
| Tuna or chicken salad plate | | | | | |
| Tuna | ½ cup | ¾ cup | ¾ cup | ¾ cup | ¾ cup |
| Swiss cheese | ½ oz | ½ oz | ½ oz | ½ oz | ½ oz |
| Mayonnaise | 2 tsp | 1 tbsp | 1 tbsp | 1 tbsp | 1 tbsp |
| Lettuce | * | * | * | * | * |
| Carrot sticks | 3 | 3 | 3 | 3 | 3 |
| Tomato wedges | 2 | 2 | 2 | 2 | 2 |
| Dill pickle | 1 | 1 | 1 | 1 | 1 |
| Potato salad | None | None | ½ cup | ½ cup | ½ cup |
| Hard roll | 1 | 1 | 1 | 1 | 1 |
| Peach | 1 medium | 1 medium | 1 medium | 1 medium | 1 medium |
| Lemon-lime soda | None | None | None | None | 12 fl oz |
| Coffee, regular or decaffeinated | * | * | * | * | * |

| Dinner | | | | | |
|---|---|---|---|---|---|
| • Ham Risotto | 1 serving | 1 serving | 1 serving | 1½ servings | 1½ servings |
| Italian green beans | ½ cup | ½ cup | ½ cup | ½ cup | ½ cup |
| Mixed green salad | 1 cup | 1 cup | 1 cup | 1 cup | 1 cup |
| Salad dressing | Low-calorie, 1 tbsp | Low-calorie, 1 tbsp | Regular, 1 tbsp | Regular, 1 tbsp | Regular, 1 tbsp |
| Muffin | None | None | None | None | 1 |
| Butter | None | None | None | None | 1 tsp |
| Fresh strawberries | ¾ cup | ¾ cup | ¾ cup | ¾ cup | ¾ cup |
| Frozen whipped topping | 1 tbsp | 2 tbsp | 2 tbsp | 2 tbsp | 2 tbsp |
| Coffee, regular or decaffeinated | * | * | * | * | * |
| **Snack** | | | | | |
| Frozen pudding on a stick | 1 | 1 | 1 | 1 | 1 |
| Popcorn | 1½ cups | 3 cups | 3 cups | 3 cups | 3 cups |
| Sugar free iced tea | * | * | * | * | * |
| Bloody Mary cocktail | | | | | |
| Vodka | None | None | None | 1 fl oz | 1 fl oz |
| Tomato juice | None | None | None | 1 cup | 1 cup |

*As desired
• Recipe on page 238

## Day Thirteen—Saturday

**ADULTS**

| | 1200 Calories | 1500 Calories | 1800 Calories | 2100 Calories | 2400 Calories |
|---|---|---|---|---|---|
| **Breakfast** | | | | | |
| Grapefruit | ½ small | ½ small | ½ small | ½ small | ½ small |
| Rye toast | 1 slice | 1 slice | 1 slice | 2 slices | 2 slices |
| Butter | None | 1 tsp | 1 tsp | 2 tsp | 2 tsp |
| Scrambled egg | 1 | | | | 1 |
| Milk | Skim or 1% lowfat, 1 cup | Skim or 1% lowfat, 1 cup | Skim or 1% lowfat, 1 cup | 2% lowfat, 1 cup | 2% lowfat, 1 cup |
| Coffee, regular or decaffeinated | * | * | * | * | * |
| **Lunch** | | | | | |
| Hero sandwich | | | | | |
| Hard roll | 1 | 1 | 1 | 1 | 1 |
| 95% fat-free ham | 2 oz | 2 oz | 2 oz | 2 oz | 2 oz |
| Beef cotto salami | 1 oz | 1 oz | 1 oz | 1 oz | 1 oz |
| Provolone cheese | ¼ oz | ¼ oz | ¼ oz | ¼ oz | ¼ oz |
| Lettuce, tomatoes, peppers | 1 cup | 1 cup | 1 cup | 1 cup | 1 cup |
| Oil | 1 tsp | 1 tsp | 1 tsp | 1 tsp | 1 tsp |
| Corn chips | None | None | ¾ oz | ¾ oz | ¾ oz |
| Plums | 2 small | 2 small | 2 small | 2 small | 2 small |
| Coffee, regular or decaffeinated | * | * | * | * | * |
| **Dinner** | | | | | |
| London broil | 2 oz | 3 oz | 3 oz | 5 oz | 5 oz |
| Baked potato | ½ med or 1 small | ½ med or 1 small | 1 medium | 1 large | 1 large |
| Yogurt | 1 tbsp | None | None | None | None |
| Sour cream | None | 1 tbsp | 2 tbsp | 2 tbsp | 2 tbsp |

| | | | | |
|---|---|---|---|---|
| Brussels sprouts | ½ cup | ½ cup | ½ cup | ½ cup |
| Sliced tomato and red onion salad | ½ cup | ½ cup | ½ cup | ½ cup |
| Italian salad dressing | Low-calorie, 1 tbsp | Regular, 2 tsp | Regular, 2 tsp | Regular, 2 tsp |
| •Chocolate Cheesecake | ¹⁄₁₂ cake | ¹⁄₁₂ cake | ¹⁄₁₂ cake | ¹⁄₁₂ cake |
| Coffee, regular or decaffeinated | * | * | * | * |
| *Snacks* | | | | |
| Orange | 1 small | 1 small | 1 large | 1 large |
| Fruit flavor sugar-free soft drink | 1 cup | 1 cup | 1 cup | 1 cup |
| Made with club soda | * | * | * | * |
| Saltines | None | 3 | 3 | 6 |
| Peanut butter | None | 1 tbsp | 1 tbsp | 2 tbsp |
| Beer | None | None | None | 12 fl oz |

*As desired
•Recipe on page 268

## Day Fourteen—Sunday

**ADULTS**

| | 1200 Calories | 1500 Calories | 1800 Calories | 2100 Calories | 2400 Calories |
|---|---|---|---|---|---|
| *Breakfast* | | | | | |
| Orange juice | ⅔ cup | ⅔ cup | ⅔ cup | ⅔ cup | ⅔ cup |
| French toast | 1 slice | 2 slices | 2 slices | 2 slices | 3 slices |
| Pancake and waffle syrup | 1 tbsp | 2 tbsp | 2 tbsp | 2 tbsp | 3 tbsp |
| Canadian style bacon | 1-oz slice | 1-oz slice | 1-oz slice | 1-oz slice | 1-oz slice |
| Milk | Skim or 1% lowfat, 1 cup | Skim or 1% lowfat, 1 cup | Skim or 1% lowfat, 1 cup | 2% lowfat, 1 cup | 2% lowfat, 1 cup |
| Coffee, regular or decaffeinated | * | * | * | * | * |
| *Dinner* | | | | | |
| Roast turkey breast | 3 oz | 3 oz | 3 oz | 4½ oz | 4½ oz |
| Gravy | None | None | None | 2 tbsp | 2 tbsp |
| Orange-cranberry relish | 1 tbsp | 1 tbsp | 1 tbsp | 2 tbsp | ⅓ cup |
| Stuffing with water chestnuts | ½ cup | ½ cup | ½ cup | ½ cup | ½ cup |
| Asparagus spears | 6–8 spears | 6–8 spears | 6–8 spears | 6–8 spears | 6–8 spears |
| Lettuce and Belgian endive salad | 2 cups | 2 cups | 2 cups | 2 cups | 2 cups |
| Salad dressing | Low-calorie, 1 tbsp | Low-calorie, 1 tbsp | Regular, 1 tbsp | Regular, 1 tbsp | Regular, 1 tbsp |
| Dinner roll | None | None | None | 1 small | 1 small |
| Butter | None | None | None | 1 tsp | 1 tsp |
| •Strawberry Bavarian | ½ cup | ½ cup | ½ cup | ½ cup | ½ cup |
| Coffee, regular or decaffeinated | * | * | * | * | * |

| | | | | | |
|---|---|---|---|---|---|
| **Supper** | | | | | |
| Split pea with ham soup | 1 cup | 1 cup | 1½ cups | 1½ cups | 1½ cups |
| French bread | 1 slice | 1 slice | 1 slice | 1 slice | 1 slice |
| Swiss cheese | 1 oz | 1 oz | 1 oz | 1 oz | 1 oz |
| Thin sliced cucumbers | ½ cup | ½ cup | ½ cup | ½ cup | ½ cup |
| Wine vinegar | * | * | * | * | * |
| Baked apple with cinnamon | 1 small | 1 medium | 1 medium | 1 medium | 1 medium |
| Brown sugar | None | 2 tsp | 2 tsp | 2 tsp | 2 tsp |
| Coffee, regular or decaffeinated | * | * | * | * | * |
| **Snacks** | | | | | |
| Celery sticks | 4 | 4 | 4 | 4 | 4 |
| Cherry tomatoes | 2 | 2 | 2 | 2 | 2 |
| Dry white wine | None | 3 fl oz | 3 fl oz | 3 fl oz | 3 fl oz |
| Cashew nuts | None | None | 8 nuts | 10 nuts | 10 nuts |

*As desired
•Recipe on page 282

# Setpoint Menus—Specially for Adolescents

## ADOLESCENTS

### Day One—Monday

| | 1500 Calories | 1800 Calories | 2200 Calories | 2400 Calories | 2800 Calories |
|---|---|---|---|---|---|
| *Breakfast* | | | | | |
| Banana | ½ small | 1 small | 1 small | 1 small | 1 small |
| Bran flakes with raisins | ½ cup | 1 cup | 1 cup | 1 cup | 1½ cups |
| Milk | Skim or 1% lowfat, 1 cup | 2% lowfat, 1 cup | 2% lowfat, 1 cup | 2% lowfat, 1 cup | 2% lowfat, 1 cup |
| Bagel | 1 half | 1 half | 1 whole | 1 whole | 1 whole |
| Butter | 1 tsp | 1 tsp | 2 tsp | 2 tsp | 2 tsp |
| *Lunch* | | | | | |
| Cheese steak on roll | 1 | 1 | 1 | 1 | 1 |
| Hard roll | 2 oz | 4 oz | 4 oz | 4 oz | 4 oz |
| Thinly sliced beef steak | 1½ oz | 1½ oz | 1½ oz | 1½ oz | 1½ oz |
| American cheese | 1 slice | 1 slice | 1 slice | 1 slice | 1 slice |
| Sliced onion | ½ cup | ½ cup | ½ cup | ½ cup | ½ cup |
| Carrot sticks | 1 small | 1 small | 1 small | 1 large | 1 cup |
| Orange | None | 1 medium | 1 medium | 1 medium | 1 medium |
| Brownie | Skim or 1% lowfat, 1 cup | 2% lowfat, 1 cup | 2% lowfat, 1 cup | 2% lowfat, 1 cup | 2% lowfat, 1 cup |
| Milk | | | | | |

| | 1 serving | 1 serving | 1 serving | 1 serving | 2 servings |
|---|---|---|---|---|---|
| *Dinner* | | | | | |
| •Jambalaya | 1 serving | 1 serving | 1 serving | 1 serving | 2 servings |
| Lettuce wedge and | ⅙ head | ⅙ head | ⅙ head | ⅙ head | ⅙ head |
| Tomato slices | ¼ cup | ¼ cup | ¼ cup | ¼ cup | ¼ cup |
| Salad dressing | Low-calorie, 1 tbsp | Regular, 2 tsp | Regular, 1 tbsp | Regular, 1 tbsp | Regular, 1 tbsp |
| Corn muffin | None | None | None | 1 medium | 1 medium |
| Butter | None | None | None | 1 tsp | 1 tsp |
| Fresh pineapple | ½ cup | ½ cup | 1 cup | 1 cup | 1 cup |
| Soft drink | Sugar free, 12 fl oz | Sugar free, 12 fl oz | Regular, 12 fl oz | Regular, 12 fl oz | Regular, 12 fl oz |
| *Snacks* | | | | | |
| Vanilla-flavor yogurt | 1 cup | 1 cup | 1 cup | 1 cup | 1 cup |
| Peach | 1 medium | 1 medium | 1 medium | 1 medium | 1 medium |
| Small crackers | None | 3 | 6 | 6 | 9 |
| Cookies | None | 1 medium | 1 medium | 1 medium | 2 medium |

*As desired
•Recipe on page 240

**ADOLESCENTS**

## Day Two—Tuesday

| | *1500 Calories* | *1800 Calories* | *2200 Calories* | *2400 Calories* | *2800 Calories* |
|---|---|---|---|---|---|
| *Breakfast* | | | | | |
| Orange eggnog | | | | | |
| Orange juice | ⅓ cup | ⅔ cup | 1 cup | 1 cup | 1 cup |
| Egg | 1 | 1 | 1 | 1 | 1 |
| Milk | Skim or 1% lowfat, 1 cup | 2% lowfat, 1 cup | 2% lowfat, 1 cup | 2% lowfat, 1 cup | 2% lowfat, 1 cup |
| Raisin bread toast | 1 slice | 1 slice | 1 slice | 1 slice | 2 slices |
| Butter | 1 tsp | 1 tsp | 1 tsp | 1 tsp | 2 tsp |
| *Lunch* | | | | | |
| Pizza, large | ⅙ pizza | ⅓ pizza | ⅓ pizza | ⅓ pizza | ⅓ pizza |
| Mixed green salad | 1½ cups | 1½ cups | 1½ cups | 1½ cups | 1½ cups |
| Salad dressing | Low-calorie, 1 tbsp | Regular, 2 tsp | Regular, 4 tsp | Regular, 4 tsp | Regular, 4 tsp |
| Apple | 1 small | 1 small | 1 small | 1 small | 1 large |
| Carbonated soft drink | Sugar free, 12 fl oz | Sugar free, 12 fl oz | Regular, 12 fl oz | Regular, 12 fl oz | Regular, 12 fl oz |
| *Dinner* | | | | | |
| •Turkey Tarragon | 1 serving | 1 serving | 1 serving | 2 servings | 2 servings |
| Curly noodles | ½ cup | ½ cup | ½ cup | ½ cup | 1 cup |
| Broccoli spears | ½ cup | ½ cup | ½ cup | ½ cup | 1 cup |
| Carrot and celery sticks | ¾ cup | ¾ cup | ¾ cup | ¾ cup | ¾ cup |
| Strawberries | ¾ cup | ¾ cup | ¾ cup | ¾ cup | ¾ cup |
| Frozen whipped topping | None | 1½ tbsp | 3 tbsp | 3 tbsp | 3 tbsp |
| Pound cake | None | None | None | None | ¾ in. slice |

| | | | | |
|---|---|---|---|---|
| **Milk** | Skim or 1% lowfat, 1 cup | 2% lowfat, 1 cup | 2% lowfat, 1 cup | 2% lowfat, 1 cup | 2% lowfat, 1 cup |

| | | | | | |
|---|---|---|---|---|---|
| *Snacks* | | | | | |
| Sandwich | | | | | |
| Ham | 1 oz | 3 oz | 3 oz | 3 oz | 3 oz |
| Rye bread | 2 slices | 2 slices | 2 slices | 2 slices | 2 slices |
| Mustard, lettuce | * | * | * | * | * |
| Milk with | Skim or 1% lowfat, 1 cup | 2% lowfat, 1 cup | 2% lowfat, 1 cup | 2% lowfat, 1 cup | 2% lowfat, 1 cup |
| Chocolate syrup | None | 1 tbsp | 2 tbsp | 2 tbsp | 2 tbsp |
| Ice milk | 1 cup | 1 cup | 1 cup | 1 cup | 1 cup |

*As desired

•Recipe on page 252

ADOLESCENTS

## Day Three—Wednesday

| | 1500 Calories | 1800 Calories | 2200 Calories | 2400 Calories | 2800 Calories |
|---|---|---|---|---|---|
| *Breakfast* | | | | | |
| Apple juice | ⅓ cup | ⅔ cup | 1 cup | 1 cup | 1 cup |
| Grilled sandwich | | | | | |
| Rye bread | 2 slices | 2 slices | 2 slices | 2 slices | 2 slices |
| Canadian bacon | 1 oz | 2 oz | 2 oz | 2 oz | 2 oz |
| Monterey cheese | ¾ oz | ¾ oz | ¾ oz | ¾ oz | 1¼ oz |
| Butter | ½ tsp | 2 tsp | 2 tsp | 2 tsp | 2 tsp |
| Milk | Skim or 1% lowfat, ½ cup | 2% lowfat, ½ cup | 2% lowfat, ½ cup | 2% lowfat, ½ cup | 2% lowfat, ½ cup |
| *Lunch* | | | | | |
| Cottage cheese fruit plate | | | | | |
| Cottage cheese | 1% lowfat, ½ cup | Creamed, ½ cup | Creamed, 1 cup | Creamed, 1 cup | Creamed, 1 cup |
| Pineapple chunks | ¼ cup | ½ cup | ½ cup | ½ cup | ½ cup |
| Peaches | ¼ cup | ½ cup | ½ cup | ½ cup | ½ cup |
| Pear slices | ¼ cup | ½ cup | ½ cup | ½ cup | ½ cup |
| Lettuce | * | * | * | * | * |
| Hard roll | 1 small | 1 small | 1 small | 1 small | 2 small |
| Butter | None | 1 tsp | 1 tsp | 1 tsp | 1 tsp |
| Cookie | 1 medium | 1 medium | 2 medium | 2 medium | 3 medium |
| Soft drink | Sugar free, 12 fl oz | Sugar free, 12 fl oz | Sugar free, 12 fl oz | Regular, 12 fl oz | Regular, 12 fl oz |
| *Dinner* | | | | | |
| •Fruited Pork Kabob | 1 serving | 1½ servings | 1½ servings | 1½ servings | 2 servings |
| •Chinese Fried Rice | ⅔ cup | ⅔ cup | ⅔ cup | ⅔ cup | 1 cup |

| | | | | | |
|---|---|---|---|---|---|
| Spinach and mushroom salad | 2 cups | 2 cups | 2 cups | 2 cups | 2 cups |
| Salad dressing | Low-calorie, 1 tbsp | Regular, 4 tsp | Regular, 4 tsp | Regular, 4 tsp | Regular, 4 tsp |
| Baked custard with nutmeg | 1/2 cup | 1/2 cup | 3/4 cup | 3/4 cup | 3/4 cup |
| Milk | Skim or 1% lowfat, 1 cup | 2% lowfat, 1 cup | 2% lowfat, 1 cup | 2% lowfat, 1 cup | 2% lowfat, 1 cup |
| *Snacks* | | | | | |
| Crackers | None | 6 small | 6 small | 6 small | 6 small |
| Swiss cheese | 1 oz | 1 oz | 1 oz | 1 oz | 1 oz |
| Zucchini and cucumber sticks | 1 cup | 1 cup | 1 cup | 1 cup | 1 cup |
| Cranberry-apple juice | None | 1/3 cup | 1 cup | 1 cup | 1 cup |
| Club soda | * | * | * | * | * |

* As desired
• Recipes on pages 236 and 260

## ADOLESCENTS

### Day Four—Thursday

| | 1500 Calories | 1800 Calories | 2200 Calories | 2400 Calories | 2800 Calories |
|---|---|---|---|---|---|
| **Breakfast** | | | | | |
| Fruited-crunchy yogurt | | | | | |
| Blueberries | ½ cup | ½ cup | ½ cup | ½ cup | ½ cup |
| Crunchy nutlike cereal nuggets | ¼ cup | ¼ cup | ¼ cup | ¼ cup | ¼ cup |
| Yogurt | Plain, 1 cup | Vanilla, 1 cup | Vanilla, 1 cup | Vanilla, 1 cup | Vanilla, 1 cup |
| Sliced ham | 2 oz | 2 oz | 2 oz | 2 oz | 2 oz |
| Bread | None | None | None | None | 1 slice |
| Butter | None | None | None | None | 1 tsp |
| **Lunch** | | | | | |
| Macaroni and cheese | 1 cup | 1 cup | 1 cup | 1½ cups | 1½ cups |
| Tomato wedges on lettuce | ½ cup | ½ cup | ½ cup | ½ cup | ½ cup |
| Grapes | 12 | 12 | 12 | 12 | 18 |
| Iced cupcake | None | None | 1 medium | 1 medium | 1 medium |
| Milk | Skim or 1% lowfat, 1 cup. | 2% lowfat, 1 cup | 2% lowfat, 1 cup | 2% lowfat, 1 cup | 2% lowfat, 1 cup |
| **Dinner** | | | | | |
| •Chili-Beef Stuffing Bake | 1 serving | 1 serving | 1 serving | 1½ servings | 1½ servings |
| Mixed green salad | 2 cups | 2 cups | 2 cups | 2 cups | 2 cups |
| Salad dressing | Low-calorie, 1 tbsp | Regular, 1 tbsp | Regular, 1 tbsp | Regular, 1 tbsp | Regular, 1 tbsp |
| Orange sections | ½ cup | ½ cup | ½ cup | ½ cup | ½ cup |
| Milk | Skim or 1% lowfat, ½ cup | 2% lowfat, ½ cup | 2% lowfat, ½ cup | 2% lowfat, ½ cup | 2% lowfat, ½ cup |

### Snacks

| Open-face sandwich | | | | | |
|---|---|---|---|---|---|
| Whole wheat bread | None | 1 slice | 1 slice | 1 slice | 2 slices |
| Turkey roll | None | 3 slices | 3 slices | 3 slices | 3 slices |
| Process American cheese | ¾ oz | ¾ oz | ¾ oz | ¾ oz | 1½ oz |
| Mayonnaise | None | 1 tsp | 1 tsp | 1 tsp | 1 tsp |
| Carrot sticks | ¼ cup | ¼ cup | ½ cup | ½ cup | ½ cup |
| Corn chips | None | 1¼ oz | 1¼ oz | 1¼ oz | 1¼ oz |
| Soft drink | Sugar free, 12 fl oz | Sugar free, 12 fl oz | Regular, 12 fl oz | Regular, 12 fl oz | Regular, 12 fl oz |

*As desired
•Recipe on page 225

## ADOLESCENTS

### Day Five—Friday

| | 1500 Calories | 1800 Calories | 2200 Calories | 2400 Calories | 2800 Calories |
|---|---|---|---|---|---|
| *Breakfast* | | | | | |
| Pineapple juice | ⅓ cup | ⅔ cup | ⅔ cup | ⅔ cup | 1 cup |
| Pumpernickel bagel | 1 whole | 1 whole | 1 whole | 1 whole | 1 whole |
| Cream cheese | 1 tbsp | 2 tbsp | 2 tbsp | 2 tbsp | 3 tbsp |
| Milk | Skim or 1% lowfat, 1 cup | 2% lowfat, 1 cup | 2% lowfat, 1 cup | 2% lowfat, 1 cup | 2% lowfat, 1 cup |
| *Lunch* | | | | | |
| Chicken noodle soup | None | None | 1 cup | 1 cup | 1 cup |
| Bacon, lettuce and tomato sandwich | | | | | |
| Bacon | 4 strips | 4 strips | 4 strips | 4 strips | 4 strips |
| Lettuce | * | * | * | * | * |
| Tomato | 3 slices | 3 slices | 3 slices | 3 slices | 3 slices |
| Mayonnaise | Low-calorie, 1 tsp | Regular, 2 tsp | Regular, 2 tsp | Regular, 2 tsp | Regular, 2 tsp |
| White bread toast | 2 slices | 2 slices | 2 slices | 2 slices | 2 slices |
| Celery sticks | ½ cup | ½ cup | ½ cup | ½ cup | ½ cup |
| Plums | 2 small | 2 small | 2 small | 2 small | 4 small |
| Lowfat chocolate milk | 1 cup | 1 cup | 1 cup | 1 cup | 1 cup |
| *Dinner* | | | | | |
| Broiled lemon sole w/parsley | 6 oz | 6 oz | 6 oz | 6 oz | 8 oz |
| Broccoli, cauliflower, and carrots | ½ cup | ¾ cup | ¾ cup | ¾ cup | ¾ cup |
| •Mock Hollandaise Sauce | ¼ cup | ¼ cup | ¼ cup | ¼ cup | ¼ cup |

|  |  |  |  |  |  |
|---|---|---|---|---|---|
| Lettuce, watercress, and endive | 2 cups | 2 cups | 2 cups | 2 cups | 2 cups |
| Salad dressing | Low-calorie, 1 tbsp | Low-calorie, 1 tbsp | Regular, 4 tsp | Regular, 4 tsp | Regular, 4 tsp |
| Dinner roll | None | None | 1 small | 1 small | 2 small |
| Butter | None | None | 1 tsp | 1 tsp | 2 tsp |
| Pear | ½ medium | None | None | None | None |
| •Chocolate Mousse Pie | None | 1/12 pie | 1/12 pie | 1/12 pie | ⅛ pie |
| Milk | Skim or 1% lowfat, 1 cup | 2% lowfat, 1 cup | 2% lowfat, 1 cup | 2% lowfat, 1 cup | 2% lowfat, 1 cup |
| *Snacks* |  |  |  |  |  |
| Rye bread | 1 slice | 1 slice | 2 slices | 2 slices | 2 slices |
| Swiss cheese | 1 oz | 1 oz | 1 oz | 1½ oz | 1½ oz |
| Roast beef | 2 oz | 2 oz | 2 oz | 3 oz | 3 oz |
| Mayonnaise | Low-calorie, 1 tsp | Regular, 2 tsp | Regular, 2 tsp | Regular, 2 tsp | Regular, 2 tsp |
| Pear | None | ½ medium | 1 medium | 1 medium | 1 medium |
| Lemonade flavor drink | Sugar free, 12 fl oz | Sugar free, 12 fl oz | Sugar free, 12 fl oz | Regular, 12 fl oz | Regular, 12 fl oz |

*As desired

•Recipes on pages 263 and 269

**ADOLESCENTS**

## Day Six—Saturday

| | 1500 Calories | 1800 Calories | 2200 Calories | 2400 Calories | 2800 Calories |
|---|---|---|---|---|---|
| *Breakfast* | | | | | |
| Grapefruit | 1 half, small | 1 half, small | 1 half, small | 1 half, small | 1 half, small |
| Cheese omelet | | | | | |
| Egg | 1 | 1 | 1 | 1 | 2 |
| Swiss cheese | ½ oz | ½ oz | ½ oz | ½ oz | 1 oz |
| Whole wheat toast | 1 slice | 1 slice | 1 slice | 1 slice | 2 slices |
| Butter | None | 1 tsp | 1 tsp | 1 tsp | 2 tsp |
| Milk | Skim or 1% lowfat, ½ cup | 2% lowfat, ½ cup | 2% lowfat, ½ cup | 2% lowfat, ½ cup | 2% lowfat, ½ cup |
| *Lunch* | | | | | |
| •Tostado | 1 | 1 | 1 | 1½ | 2 |
| Nectarine | 1 small | 1 small | 1 small | 1 small | 1 large |
| Ice milk | 1 cup | 1 cup | 1 cup | 1 cup | 1 cup |
| • Crisp Dessert Topping | None | None | 3 tbsp | 3 tbsp | 3 tbsp |
| Cola | Sugar free, 12 fl oz | Regular, 12 fl oz | Regular, 12 fl oz | Regular, 12 fl oz | Regular, 12 fl oz |
| *Dinner* | | | | | |
| Baked half chicken breast | 3 oz | 4½ oz | 4½ oz | 4½ oz | 4½ oz |
| Zucchini, carrots, and onions | ¾ cup | ¾ cup | ¾ cup | ¾ cup | ¾ cup |
| Cranberry sauce | None | 2 tbsp | 2 tbsp | 2 tbsp | 2 tbsp |
| Tossed salad | 1½ cups | 1½ cups | 1½ cups | 1½ cups | 1½ cups |
| Salad dressing | Low-calorie, 1 tbsp | Low-calorie, 1 tbsp | Regular, 4 tsp | Regular, 4 tsp | Regular, 4 tsp |

| | | | | |
|---|---|---|---|---|
| Biscuit | 1 small | 1 small | 2 small | 2 small | 2 small |
| Butter | None | 1 tsp | 2 tsp | 2 tsp | 2 tsp |
| Fresh fruit cup | 1/2 cup | 1/2 cup | 1/2 cup | 1/2 cup | 1/2 cup |
| Whipped topping | Reduced-calorie, 2 tbsp | Regular, 3 tbsp | Regular, 3 tbsp | Regular, 3 tbsp | Regular, 3 tbsp |
| Milk | Skim or 1% lowfat, 1 cup | 2% lowfat, 1 cup | 2% lowfat, 1 cup | 2% lowfat, 1 cup | 2% lowfat, 1 cup |
| *Snacks* | | | | | |
| Popcorn sprinkled with | 3 cups | 3 cups | 3 cups | 3 cups | 3 cups |
| Parmesan cheese | 1/4 cup | 1/4 cup | 1/4 cup | 1/4 cup | 1/4 cup |
| Green pepper sticks | 1/4 cup | 3/4 cup | 3/4 cup | 3/4 cup | 3/4 cup |
| Sour cream dip | None | 2 tbsp | 2 tbsp | 2 tbsp | 2 tbsp |
| Orange juice | None | None | 2/3 cup | 2/3 cup | 1 cup |

*As desired
•Recipes on pages 249 and 287

**ADOLESCENTS**

## Day Seven—Sunday

| | 1500 Calories | 1800 Calories | 2200 Calories | 2400 Calories | 2800 Calories |
|---|---|---|---|---|---|
| *Breakfast* | | | | | |
| Cranberry-apple juice | ⅔ cup | ⅔ cup | ⅔ cup | ⅔ cup | ⅔ cup |
| Pancakes | 2 medium | 2 medium | 4 medium | 4 medium | 4 medium |
| Butter | None | 1 tbsp | 2 tsp | 2 tsp | 2 tsp |
| Maple flavor syrup | 1 tbsp | 1 tbsp | 2 tbsp | 2 tbsp | 2 tbsp |
| Milk | Skim or 1% lowfat, 1 cup | 2% lowfat, 1 cup | 2% lowfat, 1 cup | 2% lowfat, 1 cup | 2% lowfat, 1 cup |
| Coffee or tea | * | * | * | * | * |
| *Dinner* | | | | | |
| Roast beef | 3 oz | 4 oz | 4 oz | 4 oz | 6 oz |
| Gravy | None | 2 tbsp | 2 tbsp | 2 tbsp | 3 tbsp |
| Baked potato | 1 medium | 1 medium | 1 medium | 1 medium | 1 medium |
| Sour cream | 2 tbsp | 2 tbsp | 2 tbsp | 2 tbsp | 2 tbsp |
| Asparagus spears | 6–8 | 6–8 | 6–8 | 6–8 | 6–8 |
| Spinach and lettuce salad | 2 cups | 2 cups | 2 cups | 2 cups | 2 cups |
| Salad dressing | Low-calorie, 1 tbsp | Regular, 4 tsp | Regular, 4 tsp | Regular, 4 tsp | Regular, 4 tsp |
| •Zabaglione | ½ cup | ½ cup | ½ cup | ½ cup | ½ cup |
| Milk | Skim or 1% lowfat, ¾ cup | 2% lowfat, ¾ cup | 2% lowfat, ¾ cup | 2% lowfat, ¾ cup | 2% lowfat, ¾ cup |

| *Soup 'n Sandwich Supper* | | | | | |
|---|---|---|---|---|---|
| •Zucchini Soup | 1 cup | 1 cup | 1 cup | 1½ cups | 1½ cups |
| Ham sandwich | | | | | |
| 95% fat-free ham | 2 oz | 3 oz | 3 oz | 4 oz | 4 oz |
| Lettuce, mustard | * | * | * | * | * |
| Rye bread | 2 slices | 2 slices | 2 slices | 2 slices | 2 slices |
| Dill pickle | 1 small | 1 | 1 | 1 | 1 |
| Orange | 1 large | 1 large | 1 large | 1 large | 1 large |
| Milk | Skim or 1% lowfat, 1 cup | 2% lowfat, 1 cup | 2% lowfat, 1 cup | 2% lowfat, 1 cup | 2% lowfat, 1 cup |
| *Snacks* | | | | | |
| Swiss cheese | 1 oz | 1½ oz | 1½ oz | 1½ oz | 1½ oz |
| Rye crackers | 4 small | 8 small | 8 small | 8 small | 8 small |
| Apple pie | None | None | None | None | ⅛ pie |
| Vanilla ice cream | None | None | None | ½ cup | ½ cup |
| Lemon-lime drink | Sugar free, 12 fl oz | Sugar free, 12 fl oz | Regular, 12 fl oz | Regular, 12 fl oz | Regular, 12 fl oz |

*As desired
•Recipes on pages 285 and 222

## ADOLESCENTS

## Day Eight—Monday

| | 1500 Calories | 1800 Calories | 2200 Calories | 2400 Calories | 2800 Calories |
|---|---|---|---|---|---|
| *Breakfast* | | | | | |
| Apricot nectar | ⅓ cup | ⅔ cup | ⅔ cup | 1 cup | 1 cup |
| Breakfast sandwich | | | | | |
| Pita pocket | 1 small | 1 small | 1 small | 1 small | 1 small |
| Pork sausage | 1 patty | 1 patty | 1 patty | 1 patty | 1 patty |
| Muenster cheese | ¾ oz | ¾ oz | ¾ oz | ¾ oz | ¾ oz |
| Milk | Skim or 1% lowfat, 1 cup | 2% lowfat, 1 cup | 2% lowfat, 1 cup | 2% lowfat, 1 cup | 2% lowfat, 1 cup |
| *Lunch* | | | | | |
| Cheeseburger on roll | | | | | |
| Hamburger roll | 1 | 1 | 1 | 1 | 1 |
| Process American cheese | ¾ oz | ¾ oz | ¾ oz | ¾ oz | ¾ oz |
| Lean hamburger | 2 oz | 3 oz | 4 oz | 4 oz | 4 oz |
| Tomato slices | 2 | 2 | 2 | 2 | 2 |
| Lettuce, onion, mustard | * | * | * | * | * |
| Catsup | 1 tbsp | 1 tbsp | 1 tbsp | 1 tbsp | 1 tbsp |
| Coleslaw | ½ cup | ½ cup | ½ cup | ½ cup | ¾ cup |
| Peach | 1 medium | 1 medium | 1 medium | 1 medium | 1 medium |
| Soft drink | Sugar free, 12 fl oz | Sugar free, 12 fl oz | Regular, 12 fl oz | Regular, 12 fl oz | Regular, 12 fl oz |

| | | | | | |
|---|---|---|---|---|---|
| **Dinner** | | | | | |
| Vegetable juice cocktail | None | 6 fl oz | 6 fl oz | 6 fl oz | 6 fl oz |
| Baked veal cutlet | 2 oz | 3 oz | 3 oz | 4 oz | 6 oz |
| •Lemon wedges | * | * | * | * | * |
| Fettuccine | ½ cup | ½ cup | ½ cup | ¾ cup | 1 cup |
| Zucchini | ½ cup | ½ cup | ½ cup | ½ cup | ½ cup |
| Spinach and onion salad | 1½ cups | 1½ cups | 1½ cups | 1½ cups | 1½ cups |
| Salad dressing | Low-calorie, 1 tbsp | Regular, 1 tbsp | Regular, 1 tbsp | Regular, 1 tbsp | Regular, 4 tsp |
| Fruit flavor gelatin | Sugar free, ½ cup | Regular, ½ cup | Regular, ½ cup | Regular, ½ cup | Regular, ½ cup |
| Strawberries | None | ⅓ cup | ⅓ cup | ⅓ cup | ⅓ cup |
| Whipped topping | None | 1½ tbsp | 1½ tbsp | 1½ tbsp | 3 tbsp |
| Milk | Skim or 1% lowfat, 1 cup | 2% lowfat, 1 cup | 2% lowfat, 1 cup | 2% lowfat, 1 cup | 2% lowfat, 1 cup |
| **Snacks** | | | | | |
| Citrus fruit cup | ½ cup | ½ cup | ½ cup | ½ cup | 1 cup |
| Bran muffin | 1 half | 1 whole | 1 whole | 1 whole | 1 whole |
| Butter | None | 1 tsp | 1 tsp | 1 tsp | 1 tsp |
| Milk | Skim or 1% lowfat, ½ cup | 2% lowfat, ½ cup | 2% lowfat, ½ cup | 2% lowfat, ½ cup | 2% lowfat, ½ cup |
| Cookies | None | None | 2 medium | 2 medium | 3 medium |

*As desired
•Recipe on page 233

**ADOLESCENTS**

## Day Nine—Tuesday

| | 1500 Calories | 1800 Calories | 2200 Calories | 2400 Calories | 2800 Calories |
|---|---|---|---|---|---|
| *Breakfast* | | | | | |
| Grape juice | ⅓ cup | ⅓ cup | ⅔ cup | ⅔ cup | 1 cup |
| • Breakfast Cereal Bar | 1 bar | 1 bar | 1 bar | 1 bar | 1 bar |
| Milk | Skim or 1% lowfat, 1 cup | 2% lowfat, 1 cup | 2% lowfat, 1 cup | 2% lowfat, 1 cup | 2% lowfat, 1 cup |
| *Lunch* | | | | | |
| Hero sandwich | | | | | |
| Hero roll | 1 half | 1 half | 1 half | 1 half | 1 whole |
| Ham | 1 oz | 2 oz | 2 oz | 2 oz | 2 oz. |
| Salami | 1 slice | 2 slices | 2 slices | 2 slices | 2 slices |
| Provolone cheese | ¾ oz | ¾ oz | 1¼ oz | 1¼ oz | 1¼ oz |
| Lettuce, tomatoes, peppers | ¾ cup | ¾ cup | ¾ cup | ¾ cup | ¾ cup |
| Oil | None | None | 1 tsp | 1 tsp | 1 tsp |
| Celery sticks | ½ cup | ½ cup | ½ cup | ½ cup | ½ cup |
| Potato chips | None | 15 | 15 | 15 | 15 |
| Tangerine | 1 medium | 1 medium | 1 medium | 1 medium | 1 medium |
| Lowfat chocolate milk | 1 cup | 1 cup | 1 cup | 1 cup | 1 cup |
| *Dinner* | | | | | |
| • Drumsticks and Broccoli | 1 serving | 1 serving | 1 serving | 2 servings | 2 servings |
| Parsley rice | ⅓ cup | ⅔ cup | ⅔ cup | ⅔ cup | 1 cup |
| Boston lettuce and shredded carrots | 1½ cups | 1½ cups | 1½ cups | 1½ cups | 1½ cups |
| Salad dressing | Low-calorie, 1 tbsp | Regular, 1 tbsp | Regular, 1 tbsp | Regular, 1 tbsp | Regular, 1 tbsp |

| | | | | | |
|---|---|---|---|---|---|
| Biscuit | None | None | 1 small | 1 small | 2 small |
| Butter | None | None | None | None | 1 tsp |
| Cantaloupe | ¼ melon | ¼ melon | ½ melon | ½ melon | ½ melon |
| Vanilla ice cream | None | None | ½ cup | ½ cup | ½ cup |
| Milk | Skim or 1% lowfat, ½ cup | 2% lowfat, ½ cup | 2% lowfat, ½ cup | 2% lowfat, ½ cup | 2% lowfat, 1 cup |
| *Snacks* | | | | | |
| Strawberry shake Milk | Skim or 1% lowfat, ½ cup | 2% lowfat, 1 cup | 2% lowfat, 1 cup | 2% lowfat, 1 cup | 2% lowfat, 1 cup |
| Strawberries | ⅓ cup | ¾ cup | ¾ cup | ¾ cup | ¾ cup |
| Graham crackers | 2 squares | 2 squares | 2 squares | 2 squares | 4 squares |

*As desired
•Recipes on pages 291 and 229

# ADOLESCENTS

## Day Ten—Wednesday

| | 1500 Calories | 1800 Calories | 2200 Calories | 2400 Calories | 2800 Calories |
|---|---|---|---|---|---|
| **Breakfast** | | | | | |
| Banana shake | | | | | |
| Banana | ½ small | 1 small | 1 small | 1 small | 1 small |
| Milk | Skim or 1% lowfat, 1 cup | 2% lowfat, 1 cup | 2% lowfat, 1 cup | 2% lowfat, 1 cup | 2% lowfat, 1 cup |
| Toasted bagel | 1 whole | 1 whole | 1 whole | 1 whole | 1 whole |
| Jelly | 2 tsp | 2 tsp | 2 tsp | 2 tsp | 2 tsp |
| Butter | None | 1 tsp | 1 tsp | 1 tsp | 1 tsp |
| **Lunch** | | | | | |
| Tomato juice | ½ cup | ½ cup | ½ cup | ½ cup | ½ cup |
| Turkey sandwich | | | | | |
| Turkey breast | 3 oz | 4½ oz | 4½ oz | 4½ oz | 4½ oz |
| Lettuce | * | * | * | * | * |
| Mayonnaise | 1 tsp | 2 tsp | 2 tsp | 2 tsp | 2 tsp |
| White bread | 2 slices | 2 slices | 2 slices | 2 slices | 2 slices |
| Potato salad | None | None | ½ cup | ½ cup | 1 cup |
| Oatmeal cookie | 1 medium | 2 medium | 2 medium | 2 medium | 2 medium |
| Lowfat chocolate milk | 1 cup | 1 cup | 1 cup | 1 cup | 1 cup |
| **Dinner** | | | | | |
| • Easy Lasagna | 1 serving | 1 serving | 1 serving | 1 serving | 1½ servings |
| Mixed green salad with | 1½ cups | 1½ cups | 1½ cups | 1½ cups | 1½ cups |
| Hard-cooked egg, quartered | None | 1 egg | 1 egg | 1 egg | 1 egg |
| Salad dressing | Low-calorie, 1 tbsp | Low-calorie, 1 tbsp | Regular, 1 tbsp | Regular, 1 tbsp | Regular, 1 tbsp |

|  | | | | | |
|---|---|---|---|---|---|
| Garlic bread toast | None | 1 slice | 2 slices | 2 slices | 2 slices |
| Butter | None | 1 tsp | 1 tsp | 1 tsp | 1 tsp |
| Blueberries | ½ cup | ½ cup | ½ cup | ½ cup | ½ cup |
| Cheesecake | None | 1/12 cheesecake | 1/12 cheesecake | 1/12 cheesecake | 1/12 cheesecake |
| Sugar-free iced tea | 12 fl oz | 12 fl oz | 12 fl oz | 12 fl oz | 12 fl oz |
| *Snacks* | | | | | |
| Popcorn | 2 cups | 2 cups | 2 cups | 2 cups | 3 cups |
| Grape juice | ⅓ cup | ⅔ cup | 1 cup | 1 cup | 1 cup |
| Club soda | * | * | * | * | * |
| Raisins and | None | None | ¼ cup | ¼ cup | ¼ cup |
| Walnuts, whole | None | None | None | 6 medium | 6 medium |

*As desired
•Recipe on page 231

**ADOLESCENTS**

## Day Eleven—Thursday

| | 1500 Calories | 1800 Calories | 2200 Calories | 2400 Calories | 2800 Calories |
|---|---|---|---|---|---|
| *Breakfast* | | | | | |
| Pineapple chunks | ½ cup | ½ cup | ½ cup | ½ cup | ½ cup |
| Oatmeal with cinnamon | ¾ cup | ¾ cup | ¾ cup | ¾ cup | 1½ cups |
| Brown sugar | None | None | 2 tsp | 2 tsp | 2 tsp |
| Doughnut | None | 1 medium | 1 medium | 1 medium | 1 medium |
| Milk | Skim or 1% lowfat, 1 cup | 2% lowfat, 1 cup | 2% lowfat, 1 cup | 2% lowfat, 1 cup | 2% lowfat, 1 cup |
| *Lunch* | | | | | |
| Grilled ham and cheese sandwich | | | | | |
| White bread | 2 slices | 2 slices | 2 slices | 2 slices | 2 slices |
| Process American cheese | ¾ oz | ¾ oz | ¾ oz | ¾ oz | ¾ oz |
| Ham | 2 oz | 3 oz | 3 oz | 3 oz | 3 oz |
| Butter | 2 tsp | 2 tsp | 2 tsp | 2 tsp | 2 tsp |
| Corn chips | None | None | 1¼ oz | 1¼ oz | 1¼ oz |
| Carrot and green pepper sticks | ¾ cup | ¾ cup | ¾ cup | ¾ cup | ¾ cup |
| Plums | 2 small | 2 small | 2 small | 2 small | 2 small |
| Milk | Skim or 1% lowfat, 1 cup | 2% lowfat, 1 cup | 2% lowfat, 1 cup | 2% lowfat, 1 cup | 2% lowfat, 1 cup |
| *Dinner* | | | | | |
| Baked flounder | 4 oz | 6 oz | 6 oz | 6 oz | 6 oz |
| Spinach with lemon | ½ cup | ½ cup | ½ cup | ½ cup | ½ cup |
| Tomato slices on lettuce | ½ cup | ½ cup | ½ cup | ½ cup | ½ cup |
| Mayonnaise | None | 2 tsp | 2 tsp | 2 tsp | 2 tsp |

| | | | | | |
|---|---|---|---|---|---|
| Crescent roll | 1 small | 1 small | 2 small | 2 small | 2 small |
| •Trifle Treat | ½ cup | ½ cup | ¾ cup | ¾ cup | ¾ cup |
| Milk | Skim or 1% lowfat, 1 cup | 2% lowfat, 1 cup | 2% lowfat, 1 cup | 2% lowfat, 1 cup | 2% lowfat, 1 cup |
| *Snacks* | | | | | |
| Fruit and cheese | | | | | |
| Apple | ½ medium | 1 medium | 1 medium | 1 medium | 1 large |
| Swiss cheese | ½ oz | 1½ oz | 1½ oz | 1½ oz | 1½ oz |
| Crackers | 6 small | 6 small | 6 small | 6 small | 9 small |
| Vanilla yogurt | None | None | None | None | 8 oz |
| Hearty granola cereal | None | None | None | None | 1½ tbsp |
| Fudge | None | None | None | 1½ oz | 1½ oz |

*As desired
•Recipe on page 284

# ADOLESCENTS

## Day Twelve—Friday

| | 1500 Calories | 1800 Calories | 2200 Calories | 2400 Calories | 2800 Calories |
|---|---|---|---|---|---|
| *Breakfast* | | | | | |
| Grapefruit juice | ½ cup | 1 cup | 1 cup | 1 cup | 1 cup |
| Grilled sandwich | | | | | |
| White bread | 2 slices | 2 slices | 2 slices | 2 slices | 2 slices |
| Peanut butter | 2 tbsp | 2 tbsp | 2 tbsp | 2 tbsp | 2 tbsp |
| Butter | 1 tsp | 1 tsp | 2 tsp | 2 tsp | 2 tsp |
| Milk | Skim or 1% lowfat, 1 cup | 2% lowfat, 1 cup | 2% lowfat, 1 cup | 2% lowfat, 1 cup | 2% lowfat, 1 cup |
| Danish ring | None | None | None | None | ⅛ ring |
| *Lunch* | | | | | |
| Tuna salad plate | | | | | |
| Tuna | ½ cup | ½ cup | ½ cup | ½ cup | ½ cup |
| Swiss cheese | 1 oz | 1 oz | 1 oz | 1 oz | 1 oz |
| Mayonnaise | 1 tsp | 1 tsp | 2 tsp | 2 tsp | 2 tsp |
| Tomato wedges | 2 | 2 | 2 | 2 | 2 |
| Radishes, celery | ½ cup | ½ cup | ½ cup | ½ cup | ½ cup |
| Lettuce, dill pickle | * | * | * | * | * |
| Hard roll | 1 small | 1 small | 1 small | 2 small | 2 small |
| Butter | None | 1 tsp | 1 tsp | 1 tsp | 1 tsp |
| Pear | ½ medium | ½ medium | 1 medium | 1 medium | 1 large |
| Soft drink | Sugar free, 12 fl oz | Sugar free, 12 fl oz | Regular, 12 fl oz | Regular, 12 fl oz | Regular, 12 fl oz |

| Dinner | | | | |
|---|---|---|---|---|
| •Easy Beef Stew | 1 serving | 1½ servings | 1½ servings | 1½ servings | 1½ servings |
| Tossed salad | ¾ cup | 1½ cups | 1½ cups | 1½ cups | 1½ cups |
| Salad dressing | Low-calorie, 1 tbsp | Low-calorie, 1 tbsp | Regular, 1 tbsp | Regular, 1 tbsp | Regular, 1 tbsp |
| Whole wheat roll | None | 1 small | 1 small | 2 small | 2 small |
| Butter | None | 1 tsp | 1 tsp | 1 tsp | 2 tsp |
| Apricot halves | ½ cup | ½ cup | ½ cup | ½ cup | ½ cup |
| Milk | Skim or 1% lowfat, 1 cup | 2% lowfat, 1 cup | 2% lowfat, 1 cup | 2% lowfat, 1 cup | 2% lowfat, 1 cup |
| Snacks | | | | | |
| Milk | Skim or 1% lowfat, 1 cup | 2% lowfat, 1 cup | 2% lowfat, 1 cup | 2% lowfat, 1 cup | 2% lowfat, 1 cup |
| Crackers | 8 small | 8 small | 8 small | 8 small | 8 small |
| •Carrot Pudding Cake | None | ½ in. slice | ½ in. slice | ½ in. slice | 1 in. slice |
| International-style instant coffee | None | None | None | 6 fl oz | 6 fl oz |

*As desired
•Recipes on pages 230 and 267

**ADOLESCENTS**                    Day Thirteen—Saturday

|  | 1500 Calories | 1800 Calories | 2200 Calories | 2400 Calories | 2800 Calories |
|---|---|---|---|---|---|
| *Breakfast* | | | | | |
| Orange juice | ½ cup | 1 cup | 1 cup | 1 cup | 1 cup |
| Egg | 1 | 1 | 1 | 1 | 1 |
| Process American cheese | ¾ oz | ¾ oz | ¾ oz | ¾ oz | ¾ oz |
| Canadian bacon | None | 1 oz | 1 oz | 1 oz | 1 oz |
| English muffin | 1 whole | 1 whole | 1 whole | 1 whole | 1 whole |
| Milk | Skim or 1% lowfat, 1 cup | 2% lowfat, 1 cup | 2% lowfat, 1 cup | 2% lowfat, 1 cup | 2% lowfat, 1 cup |
| *Lunch* | | | | | |
| •Chicken Nuggets | 4 | 6 | 6 | 6 | 8 |
| French fries | 10 medium | 10 medium | 15 medium | 15 medium | 15 medium |
| Catsup | 1 tbsp | 1 tbsp | 1 tbsp | 1 tbsp | 1 tbsp |
| Bread 'n butter pickles | 4 slices | 4 slices | 4 slices | 4 slices | 4 slices |
| Zucchini, carrot, celery, and green pepper sticks | | | | | |
| Watermelon | 1 cup | 1 cup | 1 cup | 1 cup | 1 cup |
| Milk | 1 cup | 1 cup | 1 cup | 1 cup | 1 cup |
|  | Skim or 1% lowfat, 1 cup | 2% lowfat, 1 cup | 2% lowfat, 1 cup | 2% lowfat, 1 cup | 2% lowfat, 1 cup |
| *Dinner* | | | | | |
| Tomato juice with lemon | ½ cup | ½ cup | ½ cup | ½ cup | ½ cup |
| Roast eye round beef | 2 oz | 3 oz | 3 oz | 4 oz | 6 oz |
| Green peas | ½ cup | ½ cup | ½ cup | ½ cup | ¾ cup |

| | | | | |
|---|---|---|---|---|
| Corn muffin | 1 half | 1 whole | 1 whole | 1 whole | 1 whole |
| Butter | None | 1 tsp | 1 tsp | 1 tsp | 1 tsp |
| Sliced cucumber and onion vinaigrette | 1 cup | 1 cup | 1 cup | 1 cup | 1 cup |
| •Lemon Soufflé | ½ cup | ½ cup | ½ cup | ½ cup | ½ cup |
| Milk | Skim or 1% lowfat, 1 cup | 2% lowfat, 1 cup | 2% lowfat, 1 cup | 2% lowfat, 1 cup | 2% lowfat, 1 cup |
| *Snacks* | | | | | |
| Bing cherries | 10 | 10 | 20 | 20 | 20 |
| Ice cream soda Milk | Skim or 1% lowfat, ½ cup | 2% lowfat, ½ cup | 2% lowfat, ½ cup | 2% lowfat, ½ cup | 2% lowfat, ½ cup |
| Cream soda | Sugar free, 8 fl oz | Sugar free, 8 fl oz | Sugar free, 8 fl oz | Regular, 8 fl oz | Regular, 8 fl oz |
| Vanilla ice cream | None | ½ cup | ¾ cup | ¾ cup | ¾ cup |
| Sandwich Peanut butter | None | None | 1 tbsp | 1 tbsp | 2 tbsp |
| Jelly | None | None | 2 tsp | 2 tsp | 4 tsp |
| White bread | None | None | 1 slice | 1 slice | 2 slices |

*As desired
•Recipes on pages 224 and 275

## ADOLESCENTS

### Day Fourteen—Sunday

| | 1500 Calories | 1800 Calories | 2200 Calories | 2400 Calories | 2800 Calories |
|---|---|---|---|---|---|
| *Breakfast* | | | | | |
| Cantaloupe | ¼ melon | ¼ melon | ¼ melon | ¼ melon | ¼ melon |
| French toast | 1 slice | 2 slices | 3 slices | 3 slices | 3 slices |
| Syrup | 1 tbsp | 2 tbsp | 3 tbsp | 3 tbsp | 3 tbsp |
| Butter | None | 2 tsp | 2 tsp | 2 tsp | 2 tsp |
| Milk | Skim or 1% lowfat, 1 cup | 2% lowfat, 1 cup | 2% lowfat, 1 cup | 2% lowfat, 1 cup | 2% lowfat, 1 cup |
| *Dinner* | | | | | |
| Roast turkey, light and dark meat | 2½ oz | 5 oz | 5 oz | 5 oz | 5 oz |
| Cranberry sauce | None | 2 tbsp | 2 tbsp | ¼ cup | ⅓ cup |
| Bread stuffing | ½ cup | ½ cup | ½ cup | ¾ cup | ¾ cup |
| French green beans with mushrooms | ½ cup | ½ cup | ½ cup | ½ cup | ½ cup |
| Spinach and romaine salad | 1 cup | 1 cup | 1 cup | 2 cups | 2 cups |
| Salad dressing | Low-calorie, 1 tbsp | Low-calorie, 1 tbsp | Regular, 1 tbsp | Regular, 4 tsp | Regular, 4 tsp |
| Citrus fruit cup | ½ cup | ½ cup | ½ cup | 1 cup | 1 cup |
| Milk | Skim or 1% lowfat, 1 cup | 2% lowfat, 1 cup | 2% lowfat, 1 cup | 2% lowfat, 1 cup | 2% lowfat, 1 cup |
| *Supper* | | | | | |
| •Coney Island Weiner | 1 serving | 1 serving | 1 serving | 1 serving | 2 servings |
| Carrot and cabbage slaw | ½ cup | ¾ cup | ¾ cup | ¾ cup | ¾ cup |

| | | | | | |
|---|---|---|---|---|---|
| Banana, sliced with Fruit flavor gelatin | ½ small Sugar free, ½ cup | ½ small Sugar free, ½ cup | ½ small Regular, ½ cup | ½ small Regular, ½ cup | ½ small Regular, ½ cup |
| Milk | Skim or 1% lowfat, 1 cup | 2% lowfat, 1 cup | 2% lowfat, 1 cup | 2% lowfat, 1 cup | 2% lowfat, 1 cup |
| Chocolate syrup | None | None | 1 tbsp | 1 tbsp | 1 tbsp |
| *Snacks* | | | | | |
| Sesame crackers | 3 small | 6 small | 6 small | 6 small | 6 small |
| Swiss cheese | 1 oz | 1 oz | 1 oz | 1 oz | 1 oz |
| Sugar-free soft drink | 12 fl oz | 12 fl oz | 12 fl oz | 12 fl oz | 12 fl oz |

*As desired
•Recipe on page 228

# Setpoint Menus—Specially for Older Adults

## OLDER ADULTS

### Day One—Monday

|  | 1200 Calories | 1500 Calories | 1800 Calories | 2100 Calories |
|---|---|---|---|---|
| *Breakfast* |  |  |  |  |
| Strawberries | ¾ cup | ¾ cup | ¾ cup | ¾ cup |
| Crisp whole wheat flakes cereal | ½ cup | ½ cup | 1 cup | 1 cup |
| Cinnamon raisin toast | 1 slice | 1 slice | 1 slice | 1 slice |
| Butter | 1 tsp | 1 tsp | 1 tsp | 1 tsp |
| Milk | Skim or 1% lowfat, 1 cup | Skim or 1% lowfat, 1 cup | Skim or 1% lowfat, 1 cup | 2% lowfat, 1 cup |
| Coffee, regular or decaffeinated | * | * | * | * |
| *Dinner* |  |  |  |  |
| Broiled chicken breast | 3 oz | 3 oz | 3 oz | 6 oz |
| Mashed potato | ½ cup | ½ cup | ½ cup | ½ cup |
| Zucchini and tomato | ½ cup | ½ cup | ½ cup | ½ cup |
| Mixed green salad | 1 cup | 1 cup | 1 cup | 1 cup |
| Italian salad dressing | Low-calorie, 1 tbsp | Regular, 1 tbsp | Regular, 1 tbsp | Regular, 1 tbsp |
| Gingerbread | ⅛ cake | ⅛ cake | ⅛ cake | ⅛ cake |
| Frozen whipped topping | None | 3 tbsp | 3 tbsp | 3 tbsp |
| Coffee, regular, or decaffeinated | * | * | * | * |
| *Supper* |  |  |  |  |
| •Hearty Beef-Vegetable Soup | 1 serving | 1 serving | 1 serving | 1 serving |
| Pumpernickel bread | None | 1 slice | 1 slice | 2 slices |
| Butter | None | 1 tsp | 1 tsp | 2 tsp |
| Nectarine | 1 small | 1 medium | 1 medium | 1 medium |

| | | | | |
|---|---|---|---|---|
| Cookie | None | None | 2 medium | 3 medium |
| Coffee, decaffeinated, or tea | * | * | * | * |
| *Snacks* | | | | |
| Apple | 1 small | 1 medium | 1 medium | 1 medium |
| Vegetable juice cocktail | ½ cup | ½ cup | ½ cup | ½ cup |
| Muenster cheese | 1¼ oz | 1¼ oz | 1¼ oz | 1¼ oz |
| Stone wheat crackers | None | None | 3 medium | 3 medium |

*As desired
•Recipe on page 220

**OLDER ADULTS**

## Day Two—Tuesday

|  | 1200 Calories | 1500 Calories | 1800 Calories | 2100 Calories |
|---|---|---|---|---|
| *Breakfast* |  |  |  |  |
| Orange juice | ⅓ cup | ⅔ cup | ⅔ cup | ⅔ cup |
| Poached egg | 1 | 1 | 1 | 1 |
| Oatmeal bread toast | 1 slice | 2 slices | 2 slices | 2 slices |
| Butter | None | 1 tsp | 1 tsp | 1 tsp |
| Milk | Skim or 1% lowfat, 1 cup | Skim or 1% lowfat, 1 cup | Skim or 1% lowfat, 1 cup | 2% lowfat, 1 cup |
| Coffee, regular or decaffeinated | * | * | * | * |
| *Dinner* |  |  |  |  |
| • Far Eastern Pork Curry | 1 serving | 1 serving | 1 serving | 1 serving |
| Rice cooked in broth | ⅔ cup | ⅔ cup | ⅔ cup | ⅔ cup |
| Tomato-cucumber salad |  |  |  |  |
| Tomatoes and cucumber | 1 cup | 1 cup | 1 cup | 1 cup |
| Minced onions and parsley | 2 tbsp | 2 tbsp | 2 tbsp | 2 tbsp |
| Salad oil | 1 tsp | 1 tsp | 1 tsp | 1 tsp |
| Lemon juice | ½ tsp | ½ tsp | ½ tsp | ½ tsp |
| Cantaloupe | ¼ melon | ¼ melon | ½ melon | ½ melon |
| Ice milk | None | ½ cup | ½ cup | ½ cup |
| Coffee, regular or decaffeinated | * | * | * | * |
| *Supper* |  |  |  |  |
| Sliced ham with | 1 oz | 1 oz | 1 oz | 2 oz |
| Monterey cheese melted on | 1¼ oz | 1¼ oz | 1¼ oz | 2½ oz |
| Sprouted wheat bread toast | 1 slice | 1 slice | 1 slice | 2 slices |

| | | | | |
|---|---|---|---|---|
| Waldorf salad | | | | |
| Apple, diced | ½ medium | ½ medium | ½ medium | ½ medium |
| Celery, finely diced | ¼ cup | ¼ cup | ¼ cup | ¼ cup |
| Walnuts, chopped | None | 2 halves | 2 halves | 2 halves |
| Lettuce | 2 leaves | 2 leaves | 2 leaves | 2 leaves |
| Mayonnaise with nutmeg | Low-calorie, 2 tsp | Regular, 2 tsp | Regular, 2 tsp | Regular, 2 tsp |
| Reduced calorie pudding | ½ cup | ½ cup | ½ cup | ½ cup |
| Coffee, decaffeinated, or tea | * | * | * | * |
| *Snacks* | | | | |
| Vanilla yogurt | None | None | 1 cup | 1 cup |
| Banana | ½ small | 1 small | 1 small | 1 small |
| Sugar-free iced tea | * | * | * | * |

*As desired

•Recipe on page 232

**OLDER ADULTS**

## Day Three—Wednesday

|  | 1200 Calories | 1500 Calories | 1800 Calories | 2100 Calories |
|---|---|---|---|---|
| *Breakfast* |  |  |  |  |
| Sliced peaches | 1 medium | 1 medium | 1 medium | 1 medium |
| 40% bran flakes | ½ cup | 1 cup | 1 cup | 1 cup |
| Bagel or English muffin | 1 half | 1 half | 1 half | 1 whole |
| Cream cheese | 1½ tsp | 1½ tsp | 1½ tsp | 1 tbsp |
| Milk | Skim or 1% lowfat, 1 cup | Skim or 1% lowfat, 1 cup | Skim or 1% lowfat, 1 cup | 2% lowfat, 1 cup |
| Coffee, regular or decaffeinated | * | * | * | * |
| *Lunch* |  |  |  |  |
| • Vichyssoise Soup | 1 cup | 1 cup | 1 cup | 1 cup |
| Spinach salad |  |  |  |  |
| Fresh spinach | 1 cup | 1 cup | 1 cup | 1 cup |
| Fresh mushrooms, sliced | ½ cup | ½ cup | ½ cup | ½ cup |
| Scallion, sliced | 1 | 1 | 1 | 1 |
| Hard cooked egg, quartered | None | 2 strips | 2 strips | 2 strips |
| Crisp bacon, crumbled | Low-calorie, 1 tbsp | Low-calorie, 1 tbsp | Regular, 1 tbsp | Regular, 1 tbsp |
| Creamy dressing |  |  |  |  |
| French bread | None | None | 1-oz slice | 1-oz slice |
| Butter | None | None | 1 tsp | 1 tsp |
| Green grapes | 12 | 24 | 24 | 24 |
| Coffee, regular or decaffeinated | * | * | * | * |

| *Dinner* | | | | |
|---|---|---|---|---|
| Tomato juice cocktail | ½ cup | ½ cup | ½ cup | ½ cup |
| Broiled haddock with lemon | 4 oz | 4 oz | 4 oz | 4 oz |
| Butter | 1 tsp | 1 tsp | 1 tsp | 1 tsp |
| Parsley potato | None | ½ medium | 1 medium | 1 medium |
| Deluxe baby carrots, peas, and pearl onions | ½ cup | ½ cup | ½ cup | ½ cup |
| •Easy Rice Pudding | ½ cup | ½ cup | ½ cup | ½ cup |
| Coffee, decaffeinated, or tea | * | * | * | * |
| *Snacks* | | | | |
| Very lean sliced beef | 1 oz | 1 oz | 1 oz | 2 oz |
| Party round rye bread | 2 small slices | 2 small slices | 2 small slices | 4 small slices |
| Mayonnaise | 1 tsp | 1 tsp | 1 tsp | 2 tsp |
| Apple cider | ⅓ cup | ⅓ cup | ⅓ cup | ⅔ cup |
| Cookie | None | 1 medium | 1 medium | 1 medium |

*As desired
•Recipes on pages 221 and 271

## OLDER ADULTS

### Day Four—Thursday

|  | 1200 Calories | 1500 Calories | 1800 Calories | 2100 Calories |
|---|---|---|---|---|
| **Breakfast** |  |  |  |  |
| Stewed apricots with orange peel | 4 halves | 4 halves | 8 halves | 8 halves |
| Whole wheat toast with | 2 slices | 2 slices | 2 slices | 2 slices |
| Part skim ricotta cheese | ⅓ cup | ⅓ cup | ⅓ cup | ⅓ cup |
| Honey | 1½ tsp | 1½ tsp | 1 tbsp | 1 tbsp |
| Coffee, regular or decaffeinated | * | * | * | * |
| **Lunch** |  |  |  |  |
| Cold luncheon plate |  |  |  |  |
| Cold sliced turkey breast | 3 oz | 3 oz | 3 oz | 3 oz |
| Potato salad | None | None | ½ cup | ¾ cup |
| Cold baby carrots | ½ cup | ½ cup | ½ cup | ½ cup |
| Tomato slices | 2 slices | 2 slices | 2 slices | 2 slices |
| Lettuce | * | * | * | * |
| Mayonnaise | Low-calorie, 2 tsp | Regular, 2 tsp | Regular, 2 tsp | Regular, 2 tsp |
| Whole wheat roll | 1 small | 1 small | 2 small | 2 small |
| Fresh plums | 2 small | 2 medium | 2 medium | 2 medium |
| Coffee, regular or decaffeinated | * | * | * | * |
| **Dinner** |  |  |  |  |
| • Broiled lean loin lamb chop | 2 oz | 4 oz | 4 oz | 4 oz |
| • Easy Mideastern Pilaf | 1 serving | 1 serving | 1 serving | 1 serving |
| Whole broiled tomato with | 1 medium | 1 medium | 1 medium | 1 medium |
| Bread crumbs | None | 2 tbsp | 2 tbsp | 2 tbsp |

| | | | | |
|---|---|---|---|---|
| Minted cucumber-yogurt salad | | | | |
| Sliced cucumber | ½ cup | ½ cup | ½ cup | ½ cup |
| Plain yogurt | ⅓ cup | ⅓ cup | ⅓ cup | ⅓ cup |
| Olive oil, lemon juice | 1 tsp each | 1 tsp each | 1 tsp each | 1 tsp each |
| Mint, crushed garlic | * | * | * | * |
| Sliced banana | ½ small | 1 small | 1 small | 1 small |
| Pound cake | None | None | None | ¾ in. slice |
| Coffee, decaffeinated, or tea | * | * | * | * |
| *Snacks* | | | | |
| Fruit shake made with | | | | |
| Milk | Skim or 1% lowfat, 1 cup | Skim or 1% lowfat, 1 cup | Skim or 1% lowfat, 1 cup | 2% lowfat, 1 cup |
| Strawberries | ¾ cup | ¾ cup | ¾ cup | ¾ cup |
| Graham crackers | None | 2 | 2 | 3 |

* As desired
● Recipe on page 260

**OLDER ADULTS**

### Day Five—Friday

| | 1200 Calories | 1500 Calories | 1800 Calories | 2100 Calories |
|---|---|---|---|---|
| *Breakfast* | | | | |
| Pineapple juice | ⅓ cup | ⅓ cup | ⅓ cup | ⅔ cup |
| Hot wheat cereal | ¾ cup | 1 cup | 1 cup | 1 cup |
| Whole wheat toast | None | None | 2 slices | 2 slices |
| Butter | None | None | 2 tsp | 2 tsp |
| Milk | Skim or 1% lowfat, 1 cup | Skim or 1% lowfat, 1 cup | Skim or 1% lowfat, 1 cup | 2% lowfat, 1 cup |
| Coffee, regular or decaffeinated | * | * | * | * |
| *Lunch* | | | | |
| Ham and cheese sandwich | | | | |
| Sliced ham | 2 oz | 2 oz | 2 oz | 2 oz |
| Muenster cheese | 1¼ oz | 1¼ oz | 1¼ oz | 1¼ oz |
| Rye bread | 2 slices | 2 slices | 2 slices | 2 slices |
| Mustard | * | * | * | * |
| Green pepper strips | ½ cup | ½ cup | ½ cup | ½ cup |
| Orange, sliced | 1 small | 1 large | 1 large | 1 large |
| Coffee, regular or decaffeinated | * | * | * | * |
| *Dinner* | | | | |
| •Onion-Glazed Salmon Steak | 1 serving | 1 serving | 1 serving | 1 serving |
| Parsley new potato | 1 small | 2 small | 2 small | 3 small |
| Whole green beans with lemon | ½ cup | ½ cup | ½ cup | ½ cup |
| | * | * | * | * |

| | | | | |
|---|---|---|---|---|
| Watercress-Belgian endive salad | | | | |
| Watercress and endive | 1 cup | 1 cup | 1 cup | 1 cup |
| Fresh raw mushrooms | ¼ cup | ¼ cup | ¼ cup | ¼ cup |
| Slivered green onion | 1 tbsp | 1 tbsp | 1 tbsp | 1 tbsp |
| Herb salad dressing | Low-calorie, 1 tbsp | Low-calorie, 1 tbsp | Regular, 2 tsp | Regular, 2 tsp |
| •Poached Pear with | 1 medium | 1 medium | 1 medium | 1 medium |
| •Regal Chocolate Sauce | None | 2 tbsp | 2 tbsp | 3 tbsp |
| Coffee, decaffeinated, or tea | * | * | * | * |
| *Snacks* | | | | |
| Light beer | 8 fl oz | 8 fl oz | 8 fl oz | Regular beer 12 fl oz |
| Fresh zucchini strips | 1 cup | 1 cup | 1 cup | 1 cup |
| Dip made with | | | | |
| Cottage cheese, herbs, and onion | None | ¼ cup | ¼ cup | ¼ cup |

*As desired
•Recipes on pages 243, 279, and 288

## OLDER ADULTS

### Day Six—Saturday

| | 1200 Calories | 1500 Calories | 1800 Calories | 2100 Calories |
|---|---|---|---|---|
| *Breakfast* | | | | |
| Waffles with | 1½ small | 1½ small | 3 small | 3 small |
| Fresh blueberries | ½ cup | ½ cup | ½ cup | ½ cup |
| Powdered sugar | 2 tsp | 2 tsp | None | None |
| Maple-honey flavor syrup | None | None | 2 tbsp | 2 tbsp |
| Breakfast sausage | 1 link | 1 link | 1 link | 2 links |
| Milk | Skim or 1% lowfat, ½ cup | Skim or 1% lowfat, ½ cup | Skim or 1% lowfat, ½ cup | 2% lowfat, ½ cup |
| Coffee, regular or decaffeinated | * | * | * | * |
| *Lunch* | | | | |
| Tomato-mozzarella salad | | | | |
| Tomato slices | 1 medium | 1 medium | 1 medium | 1 medium |
| Mozzarella cheese, part skim, sliced | 1½ oz | 1½ oz | 1½ oz | 1½ oz |
| Fresh basil, parsley | * | * | * | * |
| Italian salad dressing | Low-calorie, 1 tbsp | Low-calorie, 1 tbsp | Low-calorie, 1 tbsp | Regular, 1 tbsp |
| Celery hearts | 3 small stalks | 3 small stalks | 3 small stalks | 3 small stalks |
| Black olives | None | 5 | 5 | 5 |
| Whole wheat Italian bread | 1 oz slice | 2 oz slice | 2 oz slice | 2 oz slice |
| Fresh peach | 1 medium | 1 medium | 1 medium | 1 medium |
| Coffee, regular or decaffeinated | * | * | * | * |
| *Dinner Party* | | | | |
| • Lemon Chicken | 3 oz | 3 oz | 3 oz | 3 oz |
| Parsley Almond Rice | ⅔ cup | ⅔ cup | ⅔ cup | ⅔ cup |

| | | | | |
|---|---|---|---|---|
| Asparagus spears | 6 spears | 6 spears | 6 spears | 6 spears |
| Boston lettuce with | 1 cup | 1 cup | 1 cup | 1 cup |
| Pimiento and green onion | * | * | * | * |
| Vinaigrette dressing | Low-calorie, 1 tbsp | Low-calorie, 1 tbsp | Low-calorie, 1 tbsp | Regular, 2 tsp |
| Apple with | 1 small | 1 small | 1 small | 1 medium |
| Camembert cheese | None | 1¼ oz | 1¼ oz | 1¼ oz |
| English wafer crackers | None | 3 | 3 | 3 |
| Coffee, decaffeinated, or tea | * | * | * | * |
| *Snacks* | | | | |
| Baked custard | ½ cup | ½ cup | ½ cup | ½ cup |
| Dry wine | 6 fl oz | 6 fl oz | 6 fl oz | 6 fl oz |
| Oatmeal cookie | None | None | None | 1 medium |

*As desired
•Recipe on page 241

## Day Seven—Sunday

**OLDER ADULTS**

| | 1200 Calories | 1500 Calories | 1800 Calories | 2100 Calories |
|---|---|---|---|---|
| *Breakfast* | | | | |
| Cantaloupe | ¼ melon | ¼ melon | ¼ melon | ½ melon |
| Pan-grilled 95% fat-free ham | 2 oz | 2 oz | 2 oz | 2 oz |
| Biscuit | 1 small | 1 small | 2 small | 2 small |
| Strawberry jam | 2 tsp | 2 tsp | 4 tsp | 4 tsp |
| Milk | Skim or 1% lowfat, 1 cup | Skim or 1% lowfat, 1 cup | Skim or 1% lowfat, 1 cup | 2% lowfat, 1 cup |
| Coffee, regular or decaffeinated | * | * | * | * |
| *Dinner* | | | | |
| Roast eye round beef | 3 oz | 4 oz | 4 oz | 4 oz |
| Baked potato | ½ medium | 1 medium | 1 medium | 1 medium |
| Sour cream | 1 tbsp | 2 tbsp | 3 tbsp | 3 tbsp |
| Broccoli with water chestnuts | ½ cup | ½ cup | ½ cup | ½ cup |
| Mixed green salad | 1 cup | 1 cup | 1 cup | 1 cup |
| Salad dressing | Low-calorie, 1 tbsp | Low-calorie, 1 tbsp | Regular, 2 tsp | Regular, 2 tsp |
| •Chocolate Mousse Pie | 1/12 pie | 1/12 pie | 1/12 pie | ⅙ pie |
| Coffee, regular or decaffeinated | * | * | * | * |
| *Supper* | | | | |
| •Chilled Cream of Carrot Soup | 1 cup | 1 cup | 1 cup | 1½ cups |
| Whole wheat roll | 1 small | 2 small | 2 small | 2 small |
| Swiss cheese | 1 oz | 1½ oz | 2 oz | 2 oz |
| Fresh fruit cup | ½ cup | ½ cup | ½ cup | ½ cup |
| Coffee, decaffeinated, or tea | * | * | * | * |

| | | | | |
|---|---|---|---|---|
| *Snacks* | | | | |
| Tomato juice | ½ cup | ½ cup | ½ cup | ½ cup |
| Small crackers | 3 | 6 | 6 | 6 |
| Applesauce | ½ cup | ½ cup | ½ cup | ½ cup |

*As desired
•Recipes on pages 269 and 219

**OLDER ADULTS**

## Day Eight—Monday

| | 1200 Calories | 1500 Calories | 1800 Calories | 2100 Calories |
|---|---|---|---|---|
| *Breakfast* | | | | |
| Cranberry-apple juice | ⅓ cup | ⅓ cup | ⅓ cup | ⅔ cup |
| Bran flakes with raisins | ¾ cup | ¾ cup | ¾ cup | 1¼ cups |
| Milk | Skim or 1% lowfat, 1 cup | Skim or 1% lowfat, 1 cup | Skim or 1% lowfat, 1 cup | 2% lowfat, 1 cup |
| Whole wheat toast | 1 slice | 1 slice | 2 slices | 2 slices |
| Raspberry jam | 1 tsp | 1 tsp | 2 tsp | 2 tsp |
| Coffee, regular or decaffeinated | * | * | * | * |
| *Lunch* | | | | |
| Tuna-apple salad on lettuce | | | | |
| Tuna | ½ cup | ½ cup | ½ cup | ½ cup |
| Apple, diced | ½ medium | ½ medium | ½ medium | ½ medium |
| Celery, finely diced | ¼ cup | ¼ cup | ¼ cup | ¼ cup |
| Mayonnaise | Low-calorie, 2 tsp | Regular, 2 tsp | Regular, 2 tsp | Regular, 2 tsp |
| Leaf lettuce | 2 leaves | 2 leaves | 2 leaves | 2 leaves |
| Chilled green beans | ½ cup | ½ cup | ½ cup | ½ cup |
| Sesame seed bread stick | 1 medium | 2 medium | 3 medium | 3 medium |
| Sugar-free lime flavor gelatin | ½ cup | ½ cup | ½ cup | ½ cup |
| Cookie | None | 1 medium | 2 medium | 3 medium |
| Coffee, regular or decaffeinated | * | * | * | * |
| *Dinner* | | | | |
| Sautéed veal scallops | 2 oz | 3 oz | 4 oz | 4 oz |
| Butter | 1 tsp | 1 tsp | 1½ tsp | 1½ tsp |
| •Ziti with Vegetables | 1 serving | 1 serving | 1 serving | 1 serving |

| | | | | |
|---|---|---|---|---|
| Romaine and spinach salad | 1½ cups | 1½ cups | 1½ cups | 1½ cups |
| Salad dressing | Low-calorie, 1 tbsp | Low-calorie, 1 tbsp | Low-calorie, 1 tbsp | Regular, 1 tbsp |
| Orange sections with | 1 small orange | 1 large orange | 1 large orange | 1 large orange |
| Orange flavor liqueur | None | 1 tbsp | 1 tbsp | 1 tbsp |
| Coffee, decaffeinated, or tea | * | * | * | * |
| *Snacks* | | | | |
| Hot chocolate | | | | |
| Milk | Skim or 1% lowfat, 1 cup | Skim or 1 lowfat, 1 cup | Skim or 1% lowfat, 1 cup | 2% lowfat, 1 cup |
| Chocolate syrup | 1 tbsp | 1 tbsp | 1 tbsp | 1 tbsp |
| Rye crackers | 3 small | 6 small | 6 small | 6 small |
| Lemonade flavor sugar-free drink | 8 fl oz | 8 fl oz | 8 fl oz | 8 fl oz |

*As desired
•Recipe on page 255

## OLDER ADULTS

### Day Nine—Tuesday

| | 1200 Calories | 1500 Calories | 1800 Calories | 2100 Calories |
|---|---|---|---|---|
| *Breakfast* | | | | |
| Tomato juice | ½ cup | ½ cup | ½ cup | ½ cup |
| Toasted English muffin | ½ | ½ | 1 whole | 1 whole |
| Gouda cheese | 1½ oz | 1½ oz | 1½ oz | 1½ oz |
| Canadian bacon | None | None | 1 oz | 2 oz |
| Coffee, regular or decaffeinated | * | * | * | * |
| *Dinner* | | | | |
| Beef broth | 1 cup | 1 cup | 1 cup | 1 cup |
| •Oriental Chicken with | 1 serving | 1 serving | 1 serving | 1 serving |
| Rice | ⅔ cup | ⅔ cup | ⅔ cup | ⅔ cup |
| Fresh pineapple | ½ cup | ½ cup | ½ cup | ½ cup |
| •Carrot Pudding Cake | None | ½ in. slice | ½ in. slice | ½ in. slice |
| Coffee, regular or decaffeinated | * | * | * | * |
| *Supper* | | | | |
| Fresh herb omelet | | | | |
| Whole egg plus whites | 1 egg, 2 whites | 1 egg, 2 whites | 1 egg, 2 whites | 1 egg, 2 whites |
| Chopped parsley, chives, and basil | * | * | * | * |
| Butter | 1 tsp | 1 tsp | 1 tsp | 1 tsp |
| Cherry tomatoes lightly sautéed | ½ cup | ½ cup | ½ cup | ½ cup |
| Butter and garlic | 1 tsp. | 1 tsp. | 1 tsp. | 1 tsp. |
| Toast points | 1 slice | 1 slice | 1 slice | 2 slices |
| Butter | None | None | 1 tsp | 2 tsp |
| Sliced bananas and grapes | ½ cup | ½ cup | ½ cup | ½ cup |
| with fruit flavor gelatin cubes | Sugar free, | Sugar free, | Regular, | Regular, |
| | ½ cup | ½ cup | ½ cup | ½ cup |
| Coffee, decaffeinated, or tea | * | * | * | * |

*Snacks*

| | | | | |
|---|---|---|---|---|
| Fruit shake | | | | |
| Milk | Skim or 1% lowfat, 1 cup | Skim or 1% lowfat, 1 cup | Skim or 1% lowfat, 1 cup | 2% lowfat, 1 cup |
| Banana | ½ small | ½ small | ½ small | ½ small |
| Honey | 1 tbsp | 1 tbsp | 1 tbsp | 1 tbsp |
| Bran muffin | None | 1 | 1 | 1 |
| Butter | None | None | 1 tsp | 1 tsp |
| Brandy or cordial | None | None | None | 1 fl oz |

*As desired
•Recipes on pages 244 and 267

## OLDER ADULTS

### Day Ten—Wednesday

| | 1200 Calories | 1500 Calories | 1800 Calories | 2100 Calories |
|---|---|---|---|---|
| *Breakfast* | | | | |
| Apricot nectar | ⅓ cup | ⅔ cup | ⅔ cup | ⅔ cup |
| Oatmeal cooked with cinnamon and | 1 cup | 1 cup | 1 cup | 1 cup |
| Raisins | 1 tbsp | 2 tbsp | 2 tbsp | 2 tbsp |
| Milk | Skim or 1% lowfat, 1 cup | Skim or 1% lowfat, 1 cup | Skim or 1% lowfat, 1 cup | 2% lowfat, 1 cup |
| Coffee, regular or decaffeinated | * | * | * | * |
| *Luncheon Party* | | | | |
| Dry sherry | 3 fl oz | 3 fl oz | 3 fl oz | 3 fl oz |
| •Turkey and Orange Salad on | 1 serving | 1 serving | 1 serving | 1 serving |
| Lettuce leaves | * | * | * | * |
| Crescent roll | 1 small | 1 small | 1 small | 2 small |
| Butter | None | 1 tsp | 1 tsp | 1 tsp |
| Raspberry sherbet | | ½ cup | ½ cup | ½ cup |
| •Lemon Sour Cookies | 1 cookie | 1 cookie | 2 cookies | 2 cookies |
| Coffee, decaffeinated, or tea | * | * | * | * |
| *Dinner* | | | | |
| London broil | 3 oz | 4 oz | 4 oz | 4 oz |
| Mashed potatoes | ½ cup | ½ cup | ½ cup | ½ cup |
| Cooked greens | ½ cup | ½ cup | ½ cup | ½ cup |
| Horseradish or vinegar | * | * | * | * |
| Pear half stuffed with | ½ medium | ½ medium | ½ medium | ½ medium |
| Bleu cheese | None | None | 1½ oz | 1½ oz |
| Coffee, decaffeinated, or tea | * | * | * | * |

| Snacks | | | | |
|---|---|---|---|---|
| Celery and zucchini sticks | 1 cup | 1 cup | 1 cup | 1 cup |
| Crackers | 3 small | 6 small | 6 small | 6 small |
| Peanut butter | None | None | None | 2 tbsp |
| Hot milk with | Skim or 1% lowfat, 1 cup | Skim or 1% lowfat, 1 cup | Skim or 1% lowfat, 1 cup | 2% lowfat, 1 cup |
| Honey and cinnamon | 1 tbsp | 1 tbsp | 1 tbsp | 1 tbsp |

*As desired
•Recipes on pages 258 and 276

# OLDER ADULTS

## Day Eleven—Thursday

| | 1200 Calories | 1500 Calories | 1800 Calories | 2100 Calories |
|---|---|---|---|---|
| **Breakfast** | | | | |
| Apple juice | ⅓ cup | ⅔ cup | ⅔ cup | ⅔ cup |
| Whole wheat and bran cereal with dates, raisins, and walnuts | ¾ cup | 1 cup | 1 cup | 1 cup |
| Cinnamon roll | None | None | None | 1 medium |
| Milk | Skim or 1% lowfat, 1 cup | Skim or 1% lowfat, 1 cup | Skim or 1% lowfat, 1 cup | 2% lowfat, 1 cup |
| Coffee, regular or decaffeinated | * | * | * | * |
| **Lunch** | | | | |
| • Vegetable Frittata | 1 serving | 1 serving | 1 serving | 1 serving |
| Italian bread | 1 oz slice | 2 oz slice | 2 oz slice | 2 oz slice |
| Butter | None | 1 tsp | 1 tsp | 1 tsp |
| Lettuce hearts and pimiento | 1 cup | 1 cup | 1 cup | 1 cup |
| Creamy salad dressing | Low-calorie, 1 tbsp | Regular, 2 tsp | Regular, 2 tsp | Regular, 2 tsp |
| Cantaloupe | ¼ melon | ¼ melon | ¼ melon | ¼ melon |
| Coffee, regular or decaffeinated | * | * | * | * |
| **Dinner** | | | | |
| Cranberry juice cocktail | ½ cup | ½ cup | ½ cup | ½ cup |
| Roast Cornish hen | 3 oz | 3 oz | 4½ oz | 6 oz |
| Baked winter squash with | ½ cup | ½ cup | ½ cup | ¾ cup |
| Maple flavor syrup | None | 1½ tsp | 1 tbsp | 1 tbsp |
| Italian green beans | ½ cup | ½ cup | ½ cup | ½ cup |
| Poppyseed roll | None | None | 2 small | 2 small |
| Butter | None | None | 1 tsp | 1 tsp |

| | | | | |
|---|---|---|---|---|
| Broiled grapefruit with | 1 half, small | 1 half, small | 1 half, small | 1 half, small |
| Dry sherry | 1 tbsp | 1 tbsp | 1 tbsp | 1 tbsp |
| Coffee, decaffeinated, or tea | * | * | * | * |
| *Snacks* | | | | |
| Fresh peach sundae | | | | |
| Vanilla ice cream | ¾ cup | ¾ cup | ¾ cup | ¾ cup |
| Sliced peach | 1 medium | 1 medium | 1 medium | 1 medium |
| • Crisp Dessert Topping | None | 1½ tbsp | 1½ tbsp | 1½ tbsp |
| Frozen whipped topping | None | 1½ tbsp | 1½ tbsp | 1½ tbsp |
| Fruit punch flavor sugar-free drink | * | * | * | * |

*As desired
•Recipes on pages 254 and 287

**OLDER ADULTS**

## Day Twelve—Friday

| | 1200 Calories | 1500 Calories | 1800 Calories | 2100 Calories |
|---|---|---|---|---|
| **Breakfast** | | | | |
| Fresh orange sections | 1 small orange | 1 small orange | 1 small orange | 1 large orange |
| Soft-cooked egg | 1 | 1 | 1 | 1 |
| Raisin bread toast | 1 slice | 2 slices | 2 slices | 2 slices |
| Butter | 1 tsp | 2 tsp | 2 tsp | 2 tsp |
| Milk | Skim or 1% lowfat, ½ cup | Skim or 1% lowfat, ½ cup | Skim or 1% lowfat, ½ cup | 2% lowfat, ½ cup |
| Coffee, regular or decaffeinated | * | * | * | * |
| **Lunch** | | | | |
| Sandwich | | | | |
| Lean roast beef | 2 oz | 3 oz | 3 oz | 3 oz |
| Rye bread | 2 slices | 2 slices | 2 slices | 2 slices |
| Lettuce | * | * | * | * |
| Russian dressing | Low-calorie, 1 tbsp | Low-calorie, 1 tbsp | Low-calorie, 1 tbsp | Regular, 1 tbsp |
| Macaroni salad | None | ½ cup | ½ cup | ½ cup |
| Cold steamed cauliflower florets with lemon | ½ cup | ½ cup | ½ cup | ½ cup |
| Bing cherries | 10 | 20 | 20 | 20 |
| Coffee, regular or decaffeinated | * | * | * | * |
| **Dinner** | | | | |
| •Fish Florentine | 1 serving | 1 serving | 1 serving | 1 serving |
| Curly egg noodles with parsley | ½ cup | ½ cup | ½ cup | 1 cup |
| Butter | 1 tsp | 1 tsp | 1 tsp | 2 tsp |

| | | | | |
|---|---|---|---|---|
| Deluxe whole baby carrots | ½ cup | ½ cup | ½ cup | ½ cup |
| Banana slices | ½ small | ½ small | ½ small | ½ small |
| French vanilla-flavor pudding | None | None | ½ cup | ½ cup |
| Coffee, decaffeinated, or tea | * | * | * | * |
| *Snacks* | | | | |
| Milk | Skim or 1% lowfat, ½ cup | Skim or 1% lowfat, ½ cup | Skim or 1% lowfat, ½ cup | 2% lowfat, ½ cup |
| Brownie | 1 medium | 1 medium | 1 medium | 1 medium |
| Celery sticks | ½ cup | ½ cup | ½ cup | ½ cup |
| Chive cream cheese | None | None | 1 tbsp | 2 tbsp |
| Lemon-lime flavor sugar-free drink | * | * | * | * |

* As desired

• Recipe on page 235

**OLDER ADULTS**

## Day Thirteen—Saturday

| | 1200 Calories | 1500 Calories | 1800 Calories | 2100 Calories |
|---|---|---|---|---|
| *Breakfast* | | | | |
| French toast with | 2 slices | 2 slices | 2 slices | 3 slices |
| Cinnamon-clove applesauce | ½ cup | ½ cup | ½ cup | ½ cup |
| Buttered syrup | None | None | 1 tbsp | 2 tbsp |
| Crisp bacon | 1 strip | 2 strips | 2 strips | 3 strips |
| Milk | Skim or 1% lowfat, 1 cup | Skim or 1% lowfat, 1 cup | Skim or 1% lowfat, 1 cup | 2% lowfat, 1 cup |
| Coffee, regular or decaffeinated | * | * | * | * |
| *Lunch* | | | | |
| Consommé with lemon | 1 cup | 1 cup | 1 cup | 1 cup |
| Port du Salut cheese | 1½ oz | 2 oz | 2 oz | 2 oz |
| French bread | 1 oz slice | 2 slices | 2 slices | 2 slices |
| Chilled asparagus spears | 6 spears | 6 spears | 6 spears | 6 spears |
| Sweet red pepper strips | 2 | 2 | 2 | 2 |
| Nectarine | 1 small | 1 medium | 1 medium | 1 medium |
| Coffee, regular or decaffeinated | * | * | * | * |
| *Dinner Party* | | | | |
| Filet mignon | 3 oz | 4 oz | 4 oz | 4 oz |
| Butter | 1 tsp | 1 tsp | 1 tsp | 1 tsp |
| Deglazed pan drippings with | | | | |
| Dry red wine | 1 tbsp | 1 tbsp | 1 tbsp | 1 tbsp |
| Sautéed mushrooms | ½ cup | ½ cup | ½ cup | ½ cup |
| Butter | 1 tsp | 1 tsp | 1 tsp | 1 tsp |
| •Savory Hearts of Artichokes | 1 serving | 1 serving | 1 serving | 1 serving |
| Romaine salad | 1 cup | 1 cup | 1 cup | 1 cup |

| | Low-calorie, | Low-calorie, | Regular, | Regular, |
|---|---|---|---|---|
| Cheese garlic salad dressing | 1 tbsp | 1 tbsp | 2 tsp | 2 tsp |
| Fresh strawberries with | ¾ cup | ¾ cup | ¾ cup | ¾ cup |
| •Silken Raspberry Sauce | 2 tbsp | 2 tbsp | 2 tbsp | 4 tbsp |
| Coffee, decaffeinated, or tea | * | * | * | * |
| *Snacks* | | | | |
| Red burgundy wine | 3 fl oz | 3 fl oz | 6 fl oz | 6 fl oz |
| Zucchini sticks | ½ cup | ½ cup | ½ cup | ½ cup |
| Creamy bleu cheese salad dressing | None | None | 1½ tsp | 1½ tsp |
| Cheese-flavored crackers | 3 small | 6 small | 9 small | 9 small |

*As desired
•Recipes on pages 261 and 288

**OLDER ADULTS**

## Day Fourteen—Sunday

| | 1200 Calories | 1500 Calories | 1800 Calories | 2100 Calories |
|---|---|---|---|---|
| *Breakfast* | | | | |
| Grapefruit | 1 half, small | 1 half, small | 1 half, small | 1 half, small |
| Fortified oat flakes | 1 cup | 1 cup | 1 cup | 1 cup |
| Wheatberry bread toast | None | 1 slice | 1 slice | 2 slices |
| Butter | None | 1 tsp | 1 tsp | 2 tsp |
| Milk | Skim or 1% lowfat, 1 cup | Skim or 1% lowfat, 1 cup | Skim or 1% lowfat, 1 cup | 2% lowfat, 1 cup |
| Coffee, regular or decaffeinated | * | * | * | * |
| *Dinner* | | | | |
| •Turkey Cutlet with Pear | 1 serving | 1 serving | 1 serving | 1 serving |
| Parsley rice | ⅔ cup | ⅔ cup | ⅔ cup | ⅔ cup |
| French green beans with toasted almonds | ½ cup | ½ cup | ½ cup | ½ cup |
| Mixed green salad with scallions | 1 cup | 1 cup | 1 cup | 1 cup |
| Salad dressing | Low-calorie, 1 tbsp | Low-calorie, 1 tbsp | Regular, 2 tsp | Regular, 2 tsp |
| •Zabaglione over | ½ cup | ¾ cup | ¾ cup | ¾ cup |
| Blueberries | ½ cup | ½ cup | ½ cup | ½ cup |
| Coffee, regular or decaffeinated | * | * | * | * |
| *Supper* | | | | |
| Cream of mushroom soup | None | None | None | 1 cup |
| Canadian bacon | 2 oz | 3 oz | 3 oz | 3 oz |
| Sautéed apple slices | ½ cup | ½ cup | ½ cup | ½ cup |
| Butter | 1 tsp | 1 tsp | 1 tsp | 1 tsp |
| Cinnamon or nutmeg | * | * | * | * |

| | | | | |
|---|---|---|---|---|
| Baby lima beans | ⅓ cup | ½ cup | ½ cup | ½ cup |
| Relishes—celery heart | 2 stalks | 2 stalks | 2 stalks | 2 stalks |
| ripe olives | None | 5 | 5 | 5 |
| Sugar-free raspberry flavor gelatin | ½ cup | ½ cup | None | None |
| Angel food cake | None | None | ⅛ cake | ⅛ cake |
| Coffee, decaffeinated, or tea | * | * | * | * |
| *Snacks* | | | | |
| Tomato juice with | ½ cup | ½ cup | ½ cup | ½ cup |
| Bouillon | * | * | * | * |
| Thin wheat crackers | None | 6 small | 6 small | 6 small |
| Swiss cheese | 1 oz | 1 oz | 1 oz | 1½ oz |

*As desired
•Recipes on pages 250 and 285

## Cream of Carrot Soup

*Makes 4 servings, 1 cup each.*

4 medium carrots, sliced (1 cup)
1 medium onion, sliced (¾ cup)
½ cup sliced celery
2 cups chicken broth
⅓ cup packaged enriched precooked
    rice
1 teaspoon thyme leaves
½ teaspoon salt
½ cup half-and-half

Bring carrots, onion, celery, and 1 cup broth to a boil in saucepan. Cover and simmer 15 minutes. Stir in rice. Cover, remove from heat, and let stand 5 minutes. Transfer to blender; add thyme and salt. Blend until smooth. Return to saucepan and add remaining broth and the half-and-half. Heat briefly.

*One serving equals about:*

¼ cup carrot
3 tbsp onion    } = ¾ Vegetable
2 tbsp celery

⅙ cup cooked rice = ½ Bread

2 tbsp half-and-half = 1 A Bonus

*110 Calories*

219

# Cream of Vegetable Soup

*Makes 4 servings, 1½ cups each.*

1 package (10 oz) frozen green peas
2 medium onions, sliced (1½ cups)
1 small potato, peeled and sliced (¾
    cup)
½ cup sliced celery with leaves
1 small carrot, sliced (¼ cup)
1 garlic clove
1 teaspoon salt
1 teaspoon curry powder (optional)
2 cups chicken broth
1 cup half-and-half

Place vegetables, seasonings, and 1 cup of the broth in saucepan. Bring to a boil. Cover, reduce heat, and simmer 15 minutes or until vegetables are tender. Place in blender or food processor with cutting blade. Blend until smooth. Return mixture to saucepan; add remaining broth and the half-and-half. Heat briefly.

*Note*: Soup may also be served chilled.

*One serving equals about:*

¼ pkg peas
¼ small potato    } = 1 Bread

½ medium onion
1 tbsp carrot       } = 1 Vegetable
¼ small stalk celery

¼ cup half-and-half    = 2 A Bonuses

*200 Calories*

# Hearty Beef-Vegetable Soup

*Makes 4 servings, 1¾ cups each.*

3 cups beef broth
1 can (16 oz) tomatoes

1⅔ cups diced cooked lean beef (½
    lb)
1 package (10 oz) frozen sweet corn
¾ cup packaged enriched precooked
    rice
¼ teaspoon salt
⅛ teaspoon pepper
1 tablespoon finely chopped parsley

Place all ingredients except parsley in large saucepan. Stir
to break up tomatoes. Bring to a boil over medium heat.
Cover, remove from heat, and let stand 5 minutes. Add
parsley.

*One serving equals about:*

| 2 oz cooked beef | = 1 Meat |
|---|---|
| ½ cup tomatoes | = 1 Vegetable |

⅓ cup corn
⅓ cup cooked rice   } = 2 Bread

*280 Calories*

# Vichyssoise

*Makes 4 servings, about 1 cup each.*

1 can (13¾ oz) chicken broth
2 cups thinly sliced peeled potatoes
⅓ cup chopped scallions
½ teaspoon salt
1½ teaspoons unflavored gelatin
¼ cup water
1 teaspoon butter or margarine
2 cups 1% lowfat milk

Combine broth, potatoes, scallions, and salt in saucepan.
Cook until potatoes are very soft. Meanwhile, soften gelatin in water. Add butter to potato mixture and beat with
electric mixer until smooth. Add gelatin and blend thoroughly. Stir in 1 cup of the milk. Chill. Stir in remaining
milk before serving. Sprinkle with chopped chives or additional chopped scallions if desired.

*One serving equals about:*

½ cup potatoes          = 1 Bread

½ cup 1% lowfat
    milk                = ½ Milk

¼ tsp butter          ⎫
1¼ tbsp scallions     ⎬ = Negligible
                 ⎭

*140 Calories*

# Zucchini Soup

*Makes 4 servings, 1 cup each.*

  2 cups diced zucchini
  1 can (13¾ oz) chicken broth
  1 cup sliced celery with leaves
  ½ cup water
  ½ cup sliced onion
  2 tablespoons quick-cooking tapioca
  1 garlic clove
  ½ teaspoon salt
    Dash of pepper
  ½ cup half-and-half

Combine all ingredients except half-and-half in large
saucepan; let stand 5 minutes. Cook and stir over medium
heat until mixture comes to a full boil. Reduce heat and
simmer 10 minutes, stirring occasionally. Ladle half into
blender; blend at high speed until smooth, and pour into
large bowl. Repeat with remaining zucchini mixture. Stir
in half-and-half. Chill.

*Note*: Soup may also be served hot.

*One serving equals about:*

½ cup zucchini     ⎫
¼ cup celery       ⎬ = 1 Vegetable
2 tbsp onion       ⎭

2 tbsp half-and-half   = 1 A Bonus

*90 Calories*

## Chicken with Mustard Sauce

*Makes 4 servings: 1 cutlet, and about ¼ cup sauce each.*

 2 tablespoons butter or margarine
 4 chicken breast cutlets (1 lb)
 1 cup small mushrooms or
      mushroom pieces
 ¼ cup chopped green onions
 ⅛ teaspoon salt
 1 tablespoon prepared spicy
      mustard
 ⅛ teaspoon ground thyme
 ⅓ cup half-and-half

Melt butter in skillet. Add chicken, mushrooms and onions; sprinkle with salt. Cover and simmer over medium heat 15 minutes, turning cutlets once. Place cutlets on serving platter. Stir mustard and thyme into half-and-half until smooth; pour into skillet. Heat and stir until sauce is slightly thickened; serve over chicken.

*One serving equals about:*

| | |
|---|---|
| 3 oz cooked chicken breast | = 1 Meat |
| ¼ cup mushrooms | = ¼ Vegetable |
| 1½ tsp butter | = ¾ A Bonus |
| 1½ tbsp half-and-half | = ¾ A Bonus |
| 1 tbsp green onions | = Negligible |

*210 Calories*

## Chicken Nuggets

*Makes 4 servings, 4 nuggets each.*

1 pound chicken breast cutlets
1 envelope seasoned coating mix
        for chicken—original flavor

Cut chicken into about 16 small nuggets. Coat nuggets
with seasoned coating mix as directed on package. Place
in ungreased shallow baking pan. Bake at 400° for 20
minutes.

*One serving equals about:*

3 oz cooked chicken
        breast           = 1 Meat

2 tbsp seasoned
        coating mix      = 1 Bread

*190 Calories*

## Chicken Ratatouille

*Makes 6 servings: 1 or 2 chicken pieces, and
¾ cup vegetable mixture each.*

2 tablespoons butter or margarine
1 medium eggplant, cubed
2 medium zucchini, sliced
2 medium onions, sliced
1 small garlic clove, crushed
2½ pounds cut-up chicken
1 envelope seasoned coating mix
        for chicken—barbecue style

Melt butter in 13 × 9–inch baking pan. Add vegetables
and garlic; stir to coat with butter. Bake at 350° for 10
minutes. Meanwhile, coat chicken pieces with seasoned
coating mix as directed on package. Sprinkle any remaining mix evenly over vegetables. Top with chicken pieces

and bake 50 minutes longer, or until chicken and vegetables are tender.

*One serving equals about:*

| | |
|---|---|
| 2½ oz cooked chicken | = 1 Meat |
| ⅙ medium eggplant ⅓ medium zucchini ⅓ medium onion | = 1 Vegetable |
| 1⅓ tbsp seasoned coating mix | = ½ A Bonus |
| 1 tsp butter | = ½ A Bonus |

*300 Calories*

## Chili-Beef Stuffing Bake

*Makes 6 servings, about 1 cup each.*

1¼ cups very hot water
¼ cup butter or margarine, softened
1 package (6 oz) cornbread stuffing mix
1 egg, well beaten
1 pound lean ground beef
1 can (8 oz) tomato sauce
1 can (8 oz) kidney beans
1 tablespoon chili powder
1 cup shredded cheddar cheese (4½ oz)
6 tablespoons sour cream

Combine water, butter, and contents of vegetable seasoning packet from stuffing mix in a bowl; stir until butter is melted. Add stuffing crumbs; stir until moistened. Stir in egg; let stand 5 minutes. Meanwhile, brown beef in skillet. Drain off any drippings. Add tomato sauce, undrained beans, and the chili powder to beef. Heat briefly; then let cool slightly. Evenly spread half of the stuffing mixture in an ungreased 8-inch square pan or a 9-inch quiche dish. Top with the beef, then with remaining stuffing. Bake at 350° for 30 minutes. Sprinkle with cheese and bake 3 to 5 minutes longer, or until cheese is melted. Let stand 10 to 15 minutes before serving. Cut into 6 rectangles or wedges and top with sour cream. Garnish with shredded lettuce if desired.

*One serving equals about:*

| | |
|---|---|
| 2 oz cooked beef | = 1 Meat |
| 2⅔ tbsp tomato sauce | = ½ Vegetable |
| 2⅔ tbsp kidney beans | = ½ Bread |
| ½ cup cornbread stuffing | = 1½ Bread |
| 2⅔ tbsp cheddar cheese | = ½ Milk and ½ A Bonus |
| 2 tsp butter 1 tbsp sour cream } | = 1½ A Bonuses |
| ⅙ egg | = Negligible |

*470 Calories*

## Chinese Pork

*Makes 3 servings, 1 cup each.*

9 ounces lean boneless pork loin or tenderloin
1 tablespoon oil
½ cup water
2 tablespoons dry sherry wine
1 tablespoon soy sauce
2 large garlic cloves, crushed
2 thin slices fresh ginger, minced*
1 package (10 oz) frozen Chinese-style recipe vegetables with sauce

Trim any excess fat from pork. Cut meat into ½-inch cubes. Brown pork cubes in oil in large skillet. Carefully add water, wine, and soy sauce; stir in garlic and ginger. Bring to a boil over medium heat. Cover, reduce heat, and simmer until meat is tender, about 10 minutes. Move meat to side of skillet; add frozen vegetables. Bring to a *full* boil over medium heat, separating vegetables with a fork and stirring frequently. Reduce heat; cover and simmer 2 minutes. *Always cook pork thoroughly.* Serve with Chinese noodles if desired.

*One serving equals about:*

| | |
|---|---|
| 2 oz cooked pork | = 1 Meat |
| ⅓ pkg Chinese-style vegetables | = 1 Vegetable and 1 A Bonus |
| 1 tsp oil | = ½ A Bonus |
| 2 tsp sherry | = Negligible |

*220 Calories*

*Or use ⅛ teaspoon ground ginger.

## Chinese Vegetables with Beef

*Makes 3 servings, about 1 cup each.*

1 package (10 oz) frozen Chinese-
    style crispy-textured
    vegetables with seasoning
2 tablespoons sesame oil
¾ pound lean top round or flank
    steak, thinly sliced
¼ cup sliced scallions
1 garlic clove, minced
½ medium green pepper, cut in thin
    strips
3 tablespoons water
1 tablespoon sesame seed, toasted

Remove seasoning pouch from vegetable package. Heat 1 tablespoon oil in medium skillet. Add beef a few pieces at a time; cook and stir until browned. Remove from skillet. Spread frozen vegetables, scallions, and garlic in skillet. Pour remaining oil *evenly* over vegetables and stir quickly to coat pieces. Cover and cook 2 minutes, stirring once. Add green pepper. Sprinkle with contents of seasoning pouch; add water. Cook and stir about 30 seconds to blend seasonings and coat vegetables. Return steak to skillet; stir. Sprinkle with sesame seed.

*One serving equals about:*

| | |
|---|---|
| 3 oz cooked beef | = 1½ Meat |
| ⅓ pkg Chinese-style crispy-textured vegetables | = 1 Vegetable |
| 2 tsp oil | = 1 A Bonus |
| 1 tsp sesame seed | = ¼ A Bonus |
| 1⅓ tbsp scallions ⅙ cup green pepper } | = Negligible |

*290 Calories*

## Coney Island Wieners

*Makes 4 servings: 1 wiener in roll and about ¼ cup sauce each.*

¼ pound lean ground round beef
½ medium onion, chopped
1 can (8 oz) tomato sauce
1 teaspoon chili powder
¼ teaspoon Worcestershire sauce
4 wieners
4 frankfurter rolls, split

Sauté beef and onion in skillet. Stir in tomato sauce, chili powder, and Worcestershire sauce. Add wieners. Heat and stir until mixture comes to a boil. Reduce heat and simmer 10 minutes. Set wieners in rolls; spoon on sauce.

*One serving equals about:*

| | |
|---|---|
| 1 wiener | = 1 Meat and 1 A Bonus |
| ¾ oz cooked ground round | = ½ Meat |
| ¼ cup tomato sauce<br>1 tbsp onion } | = 1 Vegetable |
| 1 frankfurter roll | = 2 Bread |

*370 Calories*

## Drumsticks and Broccoli

> *Makes 6 servings: 1 drumstick with sauce and*
> *2 or 3 broccoli spears each.*

  2 tablespoons all-purpose flour
  ¼ teaspoon salt
  ⅛ teaspoon pepper
  6 chicken drumsticks (1½ lb),
      skinned
  2 tablespoons oil
  ¼ cup water
  1 small garlic clove, minced
  1 package (10 oz) frozen deluxe
      broccoli spears
  1 tablespoon lemon juice
  1 tomato, cut in wedges

Season flour with salt and pepper. Coat drumsticks with
seasoned flour. Heat oil in large skillet. Add drumsticks
and brown evenly over high heat. Reduce heat and carefully add water and the garlic. Cover and simmer 20 to
25 minutes. Push chicken to one side of skillet. Add broccoli and bring to a *full* boil over medium-high heat, separating broccoli spears with a fork. Reduce heat, cover
and simmer 5 minutes. Arrange chicken and broccoli on
serving platter. Stir lemon juice into drippings in skillet;
spoon over chicken and broccoli. Garnish with tomato
wedges.

*One serving equals about:*

| | |
|---|---|
| 2 oz dark meat chicken | = 1 Meat |
| ⅙ pkg broccoli | = ½ Vegetable |
| 1 tsp oil | = ½ A Bonus |
| ⅙ tomato<br>1 tsp flour<br>½ tsp lemon juice | = Negligible |

*190 Calories*

## Easy Beef Stew

*Makes 4 servings, about 1 cup each.*

1 pound lean beef for stew, cut in 1-inch cubes
3 carrots, cut in 1-inch slices (1½ cups)
2 potatoes, peeled and cut in 1-inch cubes (1 cup)
2 stalks celery, cut in 1-inch slices (1 cup)
1 cup small white onions, peeled
1 can (8 oz) tomato sauce
1 small bay leaf
1 tablespoon quick-cooking tapioca
½ teaspoon salt
¼ teaspoon ground thyme
Dash of pepper

Combine all ingredients in 2-quart baking dish. Cover and bake at 300° for 2½ to 3 hours (or at 250° for 4½ to 5 hours), until beef and vegetables are tender.

*One serving equals about:*

| | |
|---|---|
| 3 oz cooked beef | = 1½ Meat |
| ⅓ cup carrot | = ¾ Vegetable |
| ¼ cup celery | = ¼ Vegetable |

¼ cup onions            = ½ Vegetable

¼ cup tomato sauce  = ¾ Vegetable

¼ cup potato            = ½ Bread

¼ tablespoon
    tapioca                = Negligible

*270 Calories*

# Easy Lasagna

*Makes 4 servings: 3 ravioli and about 1 cup sauce mixture each.*

> 2⅔ cups spaghetti sauce flavored
>         with meat
> 1 package (13 oz) frozen cheese
>         ravioli with fresh ricotta
>         cheese
> ¾ pound lean ground round beef,
>         cooked
> 6 ounces part-skim mozzarella
>         cheese, shredded
> ½ cup grated Parmesan cheese

Pour about a third of the spaghetti sauce into a 9-inch square baking dish. Arrange 9 ravioli in sauce. Sprinkle with half the beef and half of the cheeses. Evenly pour on about half of remaining spaghetti sauce. Top with remaining ravioli, sprinkle with remaining beef and cheeses, and pour remaining spaghetti sauce over all. Bake at 350° for 45 minutes.

> *One serving equals about:*
>
> 2 oz cooked ground
>     round                    = 1 Meat
>
> ⅔ cup spaghetti
>     sauce                   = 2 Vegetable
>
> 1½ oz part-skim
>     mozzarella           = 1 Milk
>     cheese

| 2 tbsp Parmesan cheese | = ½ Milk |
|---|---|
| 3 oz cheese ravioli | = 1 Bread and ½ Milk and 1 A Bonus |

*490 Calories*

# Far Eastern Pork Curry

*Makes 3 servings, 1 cup each.*

1 tablespoon oil
9 ounces lean pork cutlets, cut in strips
1 cup chicken broth
2 teaspoons cornstarch
1 teaspoon curry powder
1 package (10 oz) frozen Far Eastern–style recipe vegetables with sauce

Heat oil in medium skillet. Add pork strips. Heat and stir until meat is evenly well browned. Combine broth, cornstarch, and curry powder. Carefully add to meat in skillet and bring to a boil. Move meat to one side of skillet. Add vegetables. Bring to a *full* boil over medium heat, separating vegetables with a fork and stirring frequently. Reduce heat, cover and simmer 3 minutes. Stir with pork strips. *Always cook pork thoroughly.* Serve with rice, if desired.

*One serving equals about:*

| 2 oz cooked pork | = 1 Meat |
|---|---|
| ⅓ pkg Far Eastern-style vegetables | = 1 Vegetable and 1 A Bonus |
| 1 tsp oil | = ½ A Bonus |

*270 Calories*

# Fettuccine

*Makes 4 servings, ½ cup each.*

3 ounces narrow fettuccine or
    linguini
1½ tablespoons butter or margarine
½ cup half-and-half
½ cup grated Parmesan cheese
    Dash of pepper
    Dash of nutmeg

Cook fettuccine according to package directions; drain.
Meanwhile, melt butter in small saucepan. Add half-and-
half and heat until just hot. (Do not boil.) Place fettuccine
in warm serving bowl. Add cream sauce and half of the
grated cheese; toss until pasta is evenly coated with sauce.
Continue tossing pasta, gradually adding the pepper, nutmeg, and most of the remaining cheese. Sprinkle with rest
of cheese and serve at once.

*One serving equals about:*

| | |
|---|---|
| ½ cup cooked fettuccine | = 1 Bread |
| 2 tbsp Parmesan cheese | = ½ Milk |
| 1 tsp butter | = ½ A Bonus |
| 2 tbsp half-and-half | = 1 A Bonus |

*200 Calories*

# Fettuccine Carbonara

*Makes 3 servings, about 1 cup each.*

3 ounces fettuccine or spaghetti
6 ounces cooked ham, cubed (1 cup)
1 tablespoon butter or margarine
1 package (10 oz) frozen Italian-style recipe vegetables with sauce
½ cup water
2 eggs, slightly beaten
¼ cup whole milk
¼ cup grated Parmesan cheese

Cook fettuccine as directed on package; drain. Sauté ham in butter in skillet. Add vegetables and water. Bring to a *full* boil over medium heat, separating vegetables with a fork and stirring occasionally. Reduce heat, cover, and simmer 3 minutes. Remove from heat and stir in fettuccine. Combine eggs and milk and stir into vegetable mixture. Heat gently just until slightly thickened, about 2 minutes. Sprinkle with cheese.

*One serving equals about:*

| | |
|---|---|
| 2 oz ham | = 1 Meat |
| ⅔ egg | = ⅓ Meat |
| ½ cup cooked fettuccine | = 1 Bread |
| 1⅓ tbsp whole milk<br>1⅓ tbsp Parmesan cheese | } = ½ Milk |
| ½ cup Italian-style vegetables | = 1 Vegetable and 1 A Bonus |
| 1 tsp butter | = ½ A Bonus |

*400 Calories*

# Fish Florentine

*Makes 2 servings: 2 flounder rolls and
½ cup spinach mixture each.*

1 package (10 oz) frozen chopped
    or whole leaf spinach
2 tablespoons chopped scallions
1½ teaspoons prepared spicy mustard
¼ teaspoon salt
    Dash of pepper
¾ pound flounder or sole fillets
1½ teaspoons lemon juice
¼ cup grated Gruyère or Swiss
    cheese (2 oz)

Cook spinach according to package directions; drain well.
Return to saucepan and stir in scallions, mustard, ⅛ teaspoon salt, and the pepper. Cut each fillet lengthwise in
half; sprinkle with remaining salt and the lemon juice.
Place about 1 tablespoon spinach mixture at wide end of
each fish piece; roll up. Spoon remaining spinach mixture
into 8-inch square baking dish. Top with rolled fish, seams
down. Sprinkle with cheese. Bake at 375° for 20 minutes.

*Note*: Recipe may be doubled.

*One serving equals about:*

| | |
|---|---|
| 4 oz cooked flounder | = 1 Meat |
| ½ cup spinach | = 1 Vegetable |
| 1 oz Gruyère cheese | = 1 Milk |
| 1 tbsp scallion<br>¾ tsp mustard | } = Negligible |

*270 Calories*

# Fruited Pork Kebabs

*Makes 4 servings, 1 kebab each.*

⅓ cup orange marmalade
1 tablespoon vinegar
¾ pound pork tenderloin, cut in
    1-inch cubes
1 large onion, cut in 12 wedges
1 medium red pepper, cut in eighths
1 medium green pepper, cut in
    eighths
1 can (8 oz) pineapple chunks in
    juice, drained

Melt marmalade in small saucepan over low heat. Remove from heat and blend in vinegar. Pour over pork cubes in bowl; toss to coat all pieces. Cover and marinate in refrigerator 2 hours or overnight, stirring occasionally. Alternately thread pork, vegetables, and pineapple on 4 skewers. Brush kebabs with marinade. Broil 10 minutes. Turn kebabs, brush with marinade, and broil about 10 minutes longer. *Always cook pork thoroughly.*

*One serving equals about:*

2 oz cooked pork       = 1 Meat

¼ medium red
    pepper
¼ medium green        } = 1 Vegetable
    pepper
¼ large onion

¼ cup pineapple
    chunks              = ½ Fruit

4 tsp orange
    marmalade           = 1 A Bonus

*270 Calories*

# Ginger Beef with Stir-Fry Vegetables

*Makes 3 servings, about 1 cup each.*

1 package (10 oz) frozen Japanese-
    style crispy-textured
    vegetables with seasoning
½ pound lean chuck or flank steak,
    thinly sliced and slivered
½ teaspoon ginger*
1 tablespoon oil
3 scallions, thinly sliced
2 tablespoons water

Remove seasoning pouch from vegetable package. Sprinkle steak with ginger. Heat oil in large skillet or wok. Add scallions and sauté 1 minute. Add steak and cook just until all pink disappears. Remove from pan. Spread vegetables over surface of hot skillet; stir quickly to coat pieces with oil remaining in skillet. Cover and cook 3 minutes, stirring once. Sprinkle contents of seasoning pouch over vegetables; add water and the steak. Cook and stir about 30 seconds. Serve with hot cooked rice if desired.

*One serving equals about:*

| | |
|---|---|
| 2 oz cooked beef | = 1 Meat |
| ½ cup Japanese-style crispy-textured vegetables | = ¾ Vegetable |
| 1 tsp oil | = ½ A Bonus |

*190 Calories*

*Or use ⅛ teaspoon ground ginger.

# Ham Risotto

*Makes 4 servings, 1 cup each.*

1 slice (8-oz pkg) smoked cooked
     ham, cubed (1½ cups)
1½ cups sliced mushrooms (4 oz)
½ cup chopped onion
2 tablespoons butter or margarine
1⅔ cups (13¾-oz can) chicken broth
⅛ teaspoon crushed saffron
     (optional)
1½ cups packaged enriched
     precooked rice
¼ cup grated Parmesan cheese

Sauté ham, mushrooms, and onion in butter in skillet until lightly browned. Carefully stir in broth; add saffron and bring to a full boil. Stir in rice. Cover, remove from heat, and let stand 5 minutes. Mix lightly with a fork and sprinkle with cheese.

*One serving equals about:*

| | |
|---|---|
| 2 oz ham | = 1 Meat |
| 6 tbsp mushrooms<br>2 tbsp onion } | = ½ Vegetable |
| ⅔ cup cooked rice | = 2 Bread |
| 1 tbsp Parmesan<br>     cheese | = ¼ Milk |
| 1½ tsp butter | = ¾ A Bonus |

*290 Calories*

# Ham and Sweet Potato Bake

*Makes 2 servings: ½ ham slice with ¼ cup sauce
and ½ cup potato mixture each.*

1 slice (8-oz pkg) smoked cooked
   (95% fat-free) ham
⅔ cup sliced peeled sweet potato
½ cup sliced peeled apple
⅓ cup orange juice
3 tablespoons firmly packed brown
   sugar
1 tablespoon butter
½ teaspoon grated orange rind
⅛ teaspoon dry mustard
   Dash of ground cloves

Place ham, sweet potato, and apple in shallow baking
dish. Combine remaining ingredients in small saucepan.
Heat and stir until blended; pour over ingredients in baking dish. Bake at 350° for 20 to 25 minutes, basting frequently.

*One serving equals about:*

| | |
|---|---|
| 4 oz ham | = 1 Meat |
| ⅓ cup sweet potato | = 1¼ Bread |
| ¼ cup apple | = ½ Fruit |
| ⅙ cup orange juice | = ½ Fruit |
| 1½ tbsp sugar<br>1½ tsp butter } | = 2 A Bonuses |

*360 Calories*

# Jambalaya

*Makes 6 servings, 1⅓ cups each.*

2 tablespoons butter or margarine
½ pound chicken breast cutlets, cut
   in chunks
20 large shrimp, cleaned
1 can (16 oz) stewed tomatoes
½ cup chicken broth
¼ pound smoked cooked ham, cut
   in strips
1 garlic clove, minced
5 drops hot pepper sauce
¼ teaspoon ground thyme
⅛ teaspoon cayenne
1 package (10 oz) frozen sweet corn
1 package (9 oz) frozen French-cut
   green beans
1 cup packaged enriched precooked rice

Melt butter in large skillet. Add chicken and shrimp; cook and stir until chicken is just tender and shrimp are pink. Carefully add tomatoes and chicken broth. Stir in ham and seasonings; then add corn and beans. Bring to a *full* boil over high heat, separating vegetables with a fork and stirring frequently. Stir in rice. Cover, reduce heat, and simmer 5 minutes.

*One serving equals about:*

| | |
|---|---|
| 1 oz cooked<br>   chicken breast<br>3⅓ cooked shrimp<br>⅔ oz ham | = 1 Meat |
| ⅓ cup stewed<br>   tomatoes<br>¼ cup green beans | = 1 Vegetable |
| ¼ cup corn<br>⅓ cup cooked rice | = 1¾ Bread |
| 1 tsp butter | = ½ A Bonus |

*250 Calories*

# Lemon Chicken

*Makes 4 servings: 1 chicken cutlet with
sauce and ⅔ cup rice each.*

     2 tablespoons all-purpose flour
     ¼ teaspoon salt
     ⅛ teaspoon pepper
     4 chicken breast cutlets (1 lb)
     2 tablespoons butter or margarine
     3 tablespoons lemon juice
  1½ cups packaged enriched
          precooked rice
     ¼ cup toasted slivered almonds
     1 tablespoon chopped parsley

Season flour with salt and pepper; use to coat chicken.
Melt butter in large skillet. Add chicken and sauté until
lightly browned, turning cutlets once. Remove to serving
platter. Stir lemon juice into drippings in skillet and bring
to a simmer; pour over chicken. Meanwhile, prepare rice
as directed on package. Stir almonds and parsley into rice.
Serve with the chicken. Garnish with lemon twists and
parsley sprigs, if desired.

*One serving equals about:*

| | |
|---|---|
| 3 oz cooked chicken breast | = 1 Meat |
| ⅔ cup cooked rice | = 2 Bread |
| ½ tbsp flour | = ¼ Bread |
| ½ tbsp butter <br> 1 tbsp almonds } | = 1½ A Bonuses |

*360 Calories*

# Mexican Beef Kebabs

*Makes 4 servings, 1 kebab each.*

1 tablespoon water
1 tablespoon vinegar
1 envelope Italian salad dressing
    mix
1 teaspoon chili powder
1 tablespoon oil
⅓ cup orange juice
1 pound lean top round steak, cut
    into 12 or 16 cubes
12 large cherry tomatoes
1 large green pepper, cut into 16
    chunks
1 large onion, cut into 12 wedges

Combine water and vinegar in jar with tight-fitting lid. Add salad dressing mix and chili powder; shake well. Add oil and orange juice; shake again. Pour over meat cubes, cover, and refrigerate overnight. Drain, reserving marinade. Alternately thread meat and vegetables on 4 skewers. Broil in preheated broiler or over glowing coals 4 to 5 minutes on each side, brushing frequently with marinade.

*One serving equals about:*

| | |
|---|---|
| 3 oz cooked beef (3–4 cubes) | = 1½ Meat |
| 3 cherry tomatoes | = ¾ Vegetable |
| ¼ large green pepper | = ¼ Vegetable |
| ¼ large onion | = ½ Vegetable |
| ¾ tsp oil | = ⅓ A Bonus |
| 1⅓ tbsp orange juice | = Negligible |

*250 calories*

# Onion-Glazed Salmon Steaks

*Makes 4 servings: 1 salmon steak
and ½ cup onion sauce each.*

4 salmon steaks, ¼-inch thick (1 lb)
1 cup water
2 tablespoons chopped fresh
    dillweed*
1 bay leaf
  Dash of pepper
1 package (9 oz) frozen small
    onions with cream sauce
1 tablespoon lemon juice

Remove skin from salmon steaks. Bring water to a simmer in 10-inch skillet. Add dillweed, bay leaf, and pepper. Set salmon steaks in liquid. Cover and poach over very low heat until salmon flakes easily with a fork, about 5 minutes. Lift salmon into ovenproof serving dish; discard bay leaf. Add onions and lemon juice to poaching liquid. Bring to a *full* boil over medium-high heat, stirring occasionally. Reduce heat, cover, and simmer 2 minutes. Pour onion sauce over salmon. Place under broiler 2 to 3 minutes until onions are glazed. Serve with lemon twists and garnish with sprigs of fresh dillweed if desired.

*One serving equals about:*

3 oz cooked salmon  = 1 Meat

| ¼ pkg small onions with cream sauce | = | ½ Vegetable and 1 A Bonus |

*200 Calories*

*Or use 1 tablespoon dried dillweed.

# Oriental Chicken with Rice

*Makes 3 servings: ¾ cup chicken-vegetable
mixture and ⅔ cup rice each.*

1 tablespoon soy sauce
1 inch fresh ginger, sliced
¾ pound chicken breast cutlets,
    diced
1 tablespoon oil, butter, or
    margarine
1 package (10 oz) frozen Japanese-
    style recipe vegetables with
    sauce
1 cup packaged enriched precooked
    rice
2 tablespoons chopped pecans
1 tablespoon chopped scallion
½ teaspoon minced fresh ginger

Combine soy sauce and sliced ginger in small bowl. Add
chicken and toss to coat evenly. Let stand to marinate
about 15 minutes. Sauté chicken and sliced ginger in oil
in skillet until lightly browned and tender, about 5 minutes. Remove from skillet and discard ginger. Prepare
frozen vegetables in skillet as directed on package. In
separate saucepan prepare rice as directed on package.
Return chicken to skillet and sprinkle with pecans, scallion, and minced ginger. Serve with the rice.

*One serving equals about:*

| | |
|---|---|
| 3 oz cooked chicken breast | = 1 Meat |
| ⅔ cup cooked rice | = 2 Bread |
| ⅓ pkg Japanese-style vegetables | = 1 Vegetable and 1 A Bonus |
| 2 tsp chopped pecans 1 tsp oil | = 1 A Bonus |

*410 Calories*

# Pasta Primavera

*Makes 3 servings, about 1 cup each.*

1¼ cups pasta twists
2 cups (about ½ pkg) frozen farm-
    fresh broccoli, baby carrots,
    and water chestnuts
2 tablespoons butter or margarine
⅓ cup half-and-half
2 tablespoons white wine
½ teaspoon thyme leaves, crushed
¼ teaspoon tarragon leaves, crushed
½ cup grated Parmesan cheese

Cook pasta as directed on package; drain. Cook vegetables as directed on package, reducing simmer time to 2
minutes; drain. Melt butter in large skillet. Add half-and-
half, wine, and herbs. Cook and stir 2 to 3 minutes until
sauce is smooth. Add pasta, vegetables, and cheese; mix
lightly.

*One serving equals about:*

| | |
|---|---|
| ⅔ cup cooked pasta twists | = 1⅓ Bread |
| ½ cup farm fresh broccoli, baby carrots, and water chestnuts | = 1 Vegetable |
| ⅙ cup Parmesan cheese | = ⅔ Milk |
| 2 tsp butter 2 tbsp half-and-half | } = 2 A Bonuses |
| 2 tsp white wine | = Negligible |

*290 Calories*

# Pork Chops with Corn and Zucchini

*Makes 4 servings: 2 pork chops and about
¾ cup vegetable mixture each.*

1½ cups frozen sweet corn
2 cups sliced zucchini
2 tablespoons water
8 lean pork chops, ½-inch thick
     (1¾ lb)
1 envelope seasoned coating mix
     for pork and ribs—barbecue-
     style

Place corn, zucchini, and water in 13 × 9–inch pan. Trim excess fat from chops; then coat chops with seasoned coating mix as directed on package. Sprinkle any remaining mix evenly over vegetables in pan. Arrange chops on vegetable mixture. Bake at 350° for 30 to 35 minutes. *Always cook pork thoroughly.*

*One serving equals about:*

| | |
|---|---|
| 3 oz baked pork chop | = 1½ Meat |
| ⅓ cup sweet corn | = 1 Bread |
| ½ cup zucchini | = ½ Vegetable |
| 2 tbsp seasoned coating mix | = 1 A Bonus |

*350 Calories*

# Salmon and Toasted English Muffins

*Makes 3 servings: 1⅓ cups salmon mixture and 1 muffin each.*

> 2 tablespoons all-purpose flour
> 1½ cups whole milk
> 1 package (10 oz) frozen deluxe
>      tiny peas
> ⅓ cup half-and-half
> ¼ teaspoon salt
>     Dash of pepper
> 1 can (7¾ oz) salmon, boned and
>     flaked*
> 2 tablespoons catsup
> 3 English muffins, split and toasted

Blend flour into milk in saucepan. Add peas, half-and-half, salt and pepper. Bring to a *full* boil over medium-high heat, separating peas with a fork. Remove from heat and stir until sauce is smooth. Add salmon and catsup. Cover and simmer 5 minutes over low heat. Serve over muffins.

*One serving equals about:*

| | |
|---|---|
| 2⅔ oz salmon | = 1 Meat |
| 1 English muffin | = 2 Bread |
| ½ cup peas | = 1 Bread |
| ½ cup whole milk | = ½ Milk and ½ A Bonus |
| ⅔ tbsp flour<br>1¾ tbsp half-and-half<br>⅔ tbsp catsup } | = 1½ A Bonuses |

*410 Calories*

*Or use 1 can (7 oz) water-packed tuna, drained and flaked, or 1 can (6 oz) crab meat, flaked.

# Superb Pepper Steak

*Makes 4 servings, 1¼ cups each.*

1 tablespoon cornstarch
2 tablespoons water
2 tablespoons soy sauce
  Dash of pepper
1 pound lean sirloin or flank steak,
    cut diagonally into thin strips
1 tablespoon oil
2 medium green peppers, cut into
    strips
1 small garlic clove, crushed
1½ cups boiling water
1½ cups packaged enriched
    precooked rice

Combine cornstarch, 2 tablespoons water, soy sauce, and pepper in a bowl; stir in beef. Cover and let stand at least 1 hour to marinate. Heat oil in skillet. Add beef, green peppers, and garlic; sauté until meat is brown and peppers are crisp-tender. Add boiling water; cook and stir to loosen brown particles and bring mixture to a boil. Stir in rice. Cover, remove from heat, and let stand 5 minutes. Stir before serving.

*One serving equals about:*

| | |
|---|---|
| 3 oz cooked sirloin | = 1½ Meat |
| ½ medium green pepper | = ½ Vegetable |
| ⅔ cup cooked rice | = 2 Bread |
| ¾ tsp oil | = ⅓ A Bonus |

*370 Calories*

# Tostadas

*Makes 8 servings, 1 tostada each.*

```
   8 corn tortillas
1½ pounds lean ground beef
  ½ cup chopped onion
   1 cup bottled all-purpose or hot 'n'
        spicy–flavor barbecue sauce
   1 can (16 oz) kidney beans
   2 tablespoons tomato paste
   1 teaspoon chili powder
1½ cups shredded cheddar cheese (6 oz)
   2 cups shredded lettuce
   1 large tomato, chopped
   1 cup sour cream
  10 pitted ripe olives, sliced
   2 scallions, chopped
```

Wrap tortillas in aluminum foil. Heat at 350° for 15 minutes. Meanwhile, sauté beef and onion in skillet until meat is lightly browned. Drain off any drippings. Add barbecue sauce, undrained kidney beans, tomato paste, and chili powder. Cook and stir over medium heat 10 minutes. Spread ¾ cup meat mixture on each tortilla. Add layers of cheese, lettuce, and tomato. Top with sour cream and sprinkle with olives and scallions.

*One serving equals about:*

| | |
|---|---|
| 2 oz cooked beef | = 1 Meat |
| ¼ cup kidney beans<br>1 corn tortilla | } = 2 Bread |
| 1 tbsp onion<br>¾ tsp tomato paste<br>¼ cup lettuce<br>½ tbsp scallion<br>2½ tbsp tomato | } = ¾ Vegetable |
| 3 tbsp cheddar<br>  cheese | = ½ Milk and ½<br>A Bonus |

2 tbsp barbecue
    sauce
1–2 ripe olives          } = 1½ A Bonuses
2 tbsp sour cream

*470 Calories*


# Turkey Cutlets with Pear

*Makes 2 servings: 1 cutlet with about ⅓ cup sauce,*
*⅔ cup rice, and ½ pear each.*

1 medium pear
2 teaspoons butter or margarine
¼ cup chopped onion
2 turkey breast cutlets (8 oz)
¼ cup raisins
¼ cup chicken broth
2 tablespoons orange juice
¼ teaspoon cinnamon
¾ cup packaged enriched precooked
    rice
2 tablespoons half-and-half
1 tablespoon chopped parsley

Peel, quarter, and core pear; set aside. Melt butter in 10-inch skillet. Add onion and sauté until lightly browned. Add turkey, pear, raisins, chicken broth, orange juice, and cinnamon. Cover and poach until pear and turkey are tender, about 15 minutes. Meanwhile, prepare rice as directed on package. Arrange turkey and pear on serving platter. Stir half-and-half into liquid in skillet. Cook and stir 1 to 2 minutes until sauce is slightly thickened. Pour over turkey. Stir parsley into rice and serve with turkey.

*One serving equals about:*

3 oz cooked turkey
    breast              = 1 Meat

½ medium pear          }
2 tbsp raisins          = 2 Fruit

| 2 tbsp onion | = ¼ Vegetable |
| 2/3 cup cooked rice | = 2 Bread |
| 1 tsp butter<br>1 tbsp half-and-half | = 1 A Bonus |
| 1 tbsp orange juice | = Negligible |

*440 Calories*

# Turkey Divan

*Makes 4 servings: 3 slices turkey, ¼ package broccoli,
and about ¼ cup sauce each.*

> 1 package (10 oz) frozen broccoli
>     spears or deluxe baby
>     broccoli spears
> 1 tablespoon all-purpose flour
> ¾ cup whole milk
> 1 package (3 oz) cream cheese,
>     softened
> 1½ teaspoons Worcestershire sauce
> ¼ cup grated Parmesan cheese
> 2 packages (6 oz each) oven-roasted
>     turkey breast slices

Prepare broccoli as directed on package. Drain well and
arrange in shallow 1½-quart baking dish. Combine flour
and about 2 tablespoons of the milk in saucepan, mixing
until smooth. Add remaining milk, the cream cheese and
Worcestershire sauce. Cook and stir until sauce comes to
a boil and is thickened. Pour half the sauce over broccoli;
sprinkle with half the Parmesan cheese. Add turkey; top
with remaining sauce and cheese. Bake at 350° for 10
minutes. Then broil until lightly browned.

*One serving equals about:*

| 3 oz cooked turkey<br>breast | = 1 Meat |
| ¼ pkg broccoli<br>spears | = 1 Vegetable |

3 tbsp whole milk ⎫
1 tbsp Parmesan   ⎬  = ½ Milk and ¼
  cheese         ⎭        A Bonus

1½ tbsp cream
  cheese              = 1½ A Bonuses

*250 Calories*

# Turkey Tarragon

*Makes 4 servings: 1 slice turkey and ¼ cup sauce each.*

  ¾ pound oven-roasted turkey breast
  1 tablespoon butter or margarine
  1 tablespoon all-purpose flour
  ¾ cup whole milk
  2 tablespoons chopped scallions
  ½ teaspoon tarragon leaves
  ¼ cup sour cream

Remove and discard skin from turkey; cut meat into 4
slices and set aside. Melt butter in large skillet. Stir in
flour. Carefully add milk; then stir in scallions and tarragon. Cook and stir over medium heat until mixture
thickens and comes to a boil. Add turkey slices. Cover,
reduce heat, and simmer 10 minutes. Place turkey slices
on serving platter. Stir sour cream into sauce in skillet.
Cook and stir until just hot. (Do not boil.) Serve with
turkey.

*One serving equals about:*

3 oz cooked turkey
  breast            = 1 Meat

¾ tsp butter  ⎫
¾ tsp flour   ⎬  = 1 A Bonus
3 tbsp whole milk ⎭

1 tbsp sour cream  = ½ A Bonus

*190 Calories*

# Veal Cutlets Parmesan

*Makes 4 servings: 2 cutlets and ¼ cup sauce each.*

8 veal cutlets, ¼-inch thick (1 lb)
1 envelope seasoned coating mix
    for pork
3 ounces part skim mozzarella
    cheese
1 cup spaghetti sauce without meat

Coat veal cutlets with seasoned coating mix as directed
on package. Arrange cutlets in single layer in ungreased
shallow baking dish. Bake at 400° for 10 minutes. Sprinkle
with cheese and bake 5 minutes longer. Meanwhile, heat
spaghetti sauce. Spoon around cutlets just before serving.

*One serving equals about:*

| | |
|---|---|
| 3 oz cooked veal | = 1½ Meat |
| 2 tbsp seasoned coating mix | = 1 A Bonus |
| ¾ oz part skim mozzarella cheese | = ½ Milk |
| ¼ cup spaghetti sauce | = ¾ Vegetable |

*360 Calories*

# Vegetable Frittata

*Makes 2 servings, ½ frittata each.*

1 tablespoon butter or margarine
1 cup frozen farm-fresh cauliflower,
     green beans, and corn
⅓ cup sliced mushrooms
1 tablespoon chopped onion
¼ teaspoon ground basil
¼ teaspoon salt
  Dash of pepper
4 eggs, slightly beaten
½ cup shredded cheddar cheese (1½
     oz)
1 small tomato, seeded and cut in
     strips

Melt butter in large skillet. Add frozen vegetables, mushrooms, and onion. Cook gently until vegetables are just tender and butter is absorbed, about 3 minutes. Stir in seasonings. Pour eggs over vegetable mixture. Sprinkle with cheese and top with tomato strips. Cover and simmer over low heat until eggs are set, about 15 minutes. Garnish with parsley if desired.

*One serving equals about:*

| | |
|---|---|
| 2 eggs | = 1 Meat |
| ½ cup farm-fresh cauliflower, green beans, and corn | = ⅔ Vegetable and ⅓ Bread |
| ⅙ cup mushrooms<br>1½ tsp onion<br>½ small tomato | = ⅔ Vegetable |
| ¼ cup cheddar cheese | = ½ Milk and ½ A Bonus |
| 1½ tsp butter | = ¾ A Bonus |

*340 Calories*

# Ziti with Vegetables

*Makes 2 servings, 2 cups each.*

¾ cup ziti #2
2 teaspoons oil
½ cup sliced zucchini
½ cup mushroom quarters
1 medium tomato, coarsely diced
¼ cup chopped scallions
2 tablespoons chopped fresh basil
    leaves*
1 garlic clove, minced
2 tablespoons pignoli (pine nuts)
Dash of pepper
1 tablespoon grated Parmesan
    cheese

Cook pasta according to package directions; drain. Meanwhile, heat oil in large skillet. Add zucchini and mushrooms; sauté until tender, stirring frequently. Add tomato, scallions, basil, and garlic. Cook and stir until tomato pieces are heated; add pignoli and pepper. Add to pasta and toss gently. Sprinkle with cheese before serving.

*One serving equals about:*

¾ cup cooked ziti     = 1½ Bread

¼ cup zucchini
¼ cup mushrooms    } = ½ Vegetable

½ medium tomato
2 tbsp scallions       } = ¾ Vegetable

1 tbsp pignoli        = 1 A Bonus

1½ tsp Parmesan
    cheese            = ¼ A Bonus

1 tsp oil             = ½ A Bonus

*270 Calories*

*Or use 2 teaspoons ground basil.

# Entree Salads

## Salmon-Rice Salad Mold

*Makes 4 servings, about 1 cup each.*

1½ cups water
¼ teaspoon salt
1½ cups packaged enriched
      precooked rice
2 cans (7¾ oz each) salmon, boned
      and flaked
½ cup low-calorie mayonnaise
½ cup thinly sliced celery
½ cup finely chopped onion
¼ cup chopped dill pickle

Bring water and salt to a boil. Stir in rice. Cover, remove from heat, and let stand 5 minutes. Add remaining ingredients and mix thoroughly. Firmly pack into 3½-cup mold. (If salad is not to be unmolded, chill in a serving bowl.) Cover with waxed paper. Chill about 4 hours. Unmold. Serve with lemon wedges or slices.

*Note*: Recipe may be prepared in half quantity if desired.

*One serving equals about:*

| | |
|---|---|
| 3 oz salmon | = 1 Meat |
| ⅔ cup cooked rice | = 2 Bread |
| 2 tbsp onion<br>2 tbsp celery } | = ¼ Vegetable |
| 2 tbsp low-calorie<br>  mayonnaise | = 1 A Bonus |

*330 Calories*

# Tropical Chicken Salad

*Makes 2 entree salads, 1½ cups each.*

½ cup sour cream
1 teaspoon lemon juice
2 dozen seedless green grapes,
    halved
1 cup (5 oz) diced cooked chicken
1 cup diced celery
¼ cup flaked coconut, toasted
    Spinach leaves or dark salad
        greens
½ cup thin carrot strips

Combine sour cream and lemon juice in a bowl. Stir in grapes, chicken, celery, and 2 tablespoons of the coconut. Arrange spinach leaves on individual salad plates. Spoon on chicken mixture; sprinkle with remaining coconut. Surround chicken mixture with carrot strips.

*Note*: Recipe may be prepared in half quantity if desired.

*One serving equals about:*

| | |
|---|---|
| 2½ oz cooked chicken | = 1 Meat |
| 12 grapes | = 1 Fruit |
| ½ cup celery | = ½ Vegetable |
| ¼ cup carrot | = ½ Vegetable |
| ¼ cup sour cream | = 2 A Bonuses |
| 2 tbsp coconut | = 1 A Bonus |

*340 Calories*

# Turkey and Orange Salad

*Makes 6 servings, 1 cup each.*

1 package (10 oz) frozen deluxe
    broccoli florets
2 scallions with tops
2 cups diced cooked turkey breast
    Sections from 2 medium oranges
    (1½ cups)
1 cup chopped celery
½ cup sliced mushrooms
¼ cup mayonnaise
¼ cup plain yogurt
1 teaspoon ginger
    Dash of pepper
    Salad greens
3 tablespoons salted sunflower
    kernels

Cook broccoli as directed on package, reducing simmer time to 2 minutes; drain. Place in large bowl. Chop scallions, keeping white and green parts separate. Add turkey, orange sections, celery, mushrooms, and white part of scallions to broccoli. Combine mayonnaise, yogurt, ginger, and pepper; pour over broccoli mixture. Toss gently to coat all ingredients evenly. Arrange on salad greens. Sprinkle remaining scallions and the sunflower kernels.

*One serving equals about:*

| | |
|---|---|
| ⅓ cup cooked turkey breast | = ½ Meat |
| ¼ cup orange sections | = ½ Fruit |
| ⅙ pkg deluxe broccoli florets | = ⅔ Vegetable |
| 2 tsp scallion<br>⅙ cup celery<br>1⅓ tbsp mushrooms | = ⅓ Vegetable |
| 2 tsp mayonnaise | = 1 A Bonus |

| 1½ tsp sunflower kernels | = ½ A Bonus |
|---|---|
| 2 tsp plain yogurt | = Negligible |

*210 Calories*

# Vegetable Pasta Salad

*Makes 4 servings, about 1 cup each.*

2 cups pasta twists
2 cups frozen farm-fresh broccoli, green beans, pearl onions, and red peppers
1 cup 1% milkfat small-curd cottage cheese
1½ cups (8 oz) diced cooked ham
¼ cup whole milk
½ teaspoon ground basil
⅛ teaspoon garlic powder
⅛ teaspoon pepper

Cook pasta as directed on package; drain. Cook vegetables as directed on package, reducing simmer time to 2 minutes; drain. Place pasta and vegetables in large serving bowl. Add remaining ingredients and toss together gently. Chill.

*One serving equals about:*

| ⅔ cup cooked pasta twists | = 1¼ Bread |
|---|---|
| ½ cup vegetables | = 1 Vegetable |
| ¼ cup 1% milkfat cottage cheese | = ¼ Milk and ¼ A Bonus |
| 2 oz ham | = 1 Meat |
| 1 tbsp whole milk | = Negligible |

*300 Calories*

# Side Dishes

## Chinese Fried Rice

*Makes 4 servings, about ⅔ cup each.*

1½ cups water
1½ cups packaged enriched
    precooked rice
1 egg, beaten
¼ cup chopped scallions
3 tablespoons butter or margarine
2 tablespoons soy sauce
⅛ teaspoon garlic powder

Bring 1 cup of the water to a boil in saucepan. Stir in rice. Cover, remove from heat, and let stand 5 minutes. Meanwhile, scramble egg with scallions in butter in 10-inch skillet until egg is set. Add rice; cook and stir over medium heat until rice and scallions are lightly browned, about 5 minutes. Combine remaining water, soy sauce, and garlic powder; stir into rice mixture. Heat briefly.

*One serving equals about:*

⅔ cup cooked rice = 2 Bread

2 tsp butter = 1 A Bonus

¼ egg
1 tbsp scallion  } = ½ A Bonus

*230 Calories*

## Easy Mideastern Pilaf

*Makes 2 servings, about 1 cup each.*

2 teaspoons butter or margarine
½ medium onion, finely chopped

1½ tablespoons sliced almonds (10
  almonds)
¾ cup beef broth
2 tablespoons raisins
½ teaspoon curry powder*
¾ cup packaged enriched precooked
  rice
1 tablespoon chopped parsley

Melt butter in skillet. Add onion and almonds; cook and
stir until lightly browned. Carefully add beef broth; stir
in raisins and curry powder. Bring to a boil; stir in rice.
Cover, remove from heat, and let stand 5 minutes. Stir
in parsley just before serving.

*One serving equals about:*

| | |
|---|---|
| ⅔ cup cooked rice | = 2 Bread |
| 1 tbsp raisins | = ½ Fruit |
| ¼ medium onion | = ½ Vegetable |
| 5 almonds<br>1 tsp butter } | = 1 A Bonus |

*240 Calories*

*Or use ¼ teaspoon *each* cinnamon and cloves.

## Savory Hearts of Artichokes

*Makes 6 servings, about ½ cup each.*

2 teaspoons oil
1 package (9 oz) frozen deluxe
  artichoke hearts, thawed
1 package (10 oz) frozen green peas
  and pearl onions
1 cup chicken broth
1 bay leaf
¼ teaspoon ground tarragon
¼ teaspoon pepper

Heat oil in 10-inch skillet. Add artichoke hearts and sauté
over high heat until evenly browned, turning frequently.

Reduce heat to medium high; add peas and onions, broth, and seasonings. Bring to a *full* boil, stirring occasionally. Reduce heat to low, cover, and simmer *very gently* until vegetables are just tender, 5 to 7 minutes. Do not drain.

*One serving equals about:*

| | |
|---|---|
| ⅙ pkg artichoke hearts | = ½ Vegetable |
| ⅙ pkg peas and pearl onions | = ½ Bread |
| ⅓ tsp oil | = Negligible |

*70 Calories*

## Savory Lemon Rice

*Makes 4 servings, ⅔ cup each.*

½ garlic clove, minced
2 tablespoons butter or margarine
1½ cups chicken broth
¼ teaspoon salt
1½ cups packaged enriched
    precooked rice
2 tablespoons chopped parsley
1 tablespoon lemon juice
1 teaspoon grated lemon rind

Sauté garlic in butter in saucepan until golden brown. Carefully add broth; stir in salt. Bring quickly to a boil over high heat. Stir in rice. Cover, remove from heat, and let stand 5 minutes. Add parsley, lemon juice, and rind; mix lightly with a fork.

*One serving equals about:*

| | |
|---|---|
| 1½ tsp butter | = ¾ A Bonus |
| ⅔ cup cooked rice | = 2 Bread |

*190 Calories*

# ⅄ Sauce

## Mock Hollandaise Sauce

*Makes 1¼ cups or 5 servings.*

¾ cup water
1½ teaspoons cornstarch
1 egg
1 egg yolk
3 tablespoons lemon juice
½ teaspoon salt
Dash of cayenne

Gradually stir water into cornstarch in small saucepan. Bring to a boil; cook and stir 1 minute. Beat egg and egg yolk in bowl until light and fluffy, using wire whisk or electric mixer. Beat in lemon juice, salt, and cayenne. Gradually pour hot liquid into egg mixture, beating constantly. Return to saucepan and heat gently, beating constantly until thickened. (Do not boil.) Serve over hot cooked vegetables.

*One serving equals about:*

¼ cup sauce          = ½ A Bonus

*35 Calories*

## Apple Crisp

*Makes 8 servings, about ⅔ cup each.*

> 4 cups sliced peeled apples (4
>  medium)
> ½ cup unsifted all-purpose flour
> ½ cup firmly packed brown sugar
> ½ teaspoon cinnamon
> ¼ cup butter or margarine
> 1 cup 40% bran flakes

Arrange apple slices in 8-inch square baking dish. Combine flour, sugar, and cinnamon in bowl; cut in butter until mixture resembles coarse meal. Add cereal and toss together lightly. Sprinkle over apples. Bake at 375° for 20 to 25 minutes.

*One serving equals about:*

½ cup sliced apple    = 1 Fruit

1 tbsp flour
1 tbsp brown sugar
1½ tsp butter                = 2¼ A Bonuses
⅛ cup 40% bran
  flakes

*180 Calories*

264

# Banana Crème Brûlée

*Makes 6 servings, about ½ cup each.*

1 package (4-serving size) vanilla-
     flavor pudding and pie filling
1½ cups whole milk
1½ cups thawed frozen whipped
     topping
¼ cup firmly packed light brown
     sugar
½ teaspoon cinnamon
3 small bananas

Combine pudding mix and milk in saucepan. Cook and
stir over medium heat until mixture comes to a *full boil*.
Pour into bowl and place waxed paper directly on surface
of hot pudding. Chill. Beat slowly with rotary beater until
smooth. Fold in whipped topping. Pour into shallow 1-
quart baking dish or a 9-inch pie pan; keep chilled. Just
before serving, mix brown sugar and cinnamon. Sprinkle
over pudding. Broil about 6 inches from heat until sugar
is evenly browned. Slice bananas into individual serving
dishes and spoon pudding on top.

*One serving equals about:*

½ small banana          = 1 Fruit

¼ cup whole milk        = ¼ Milk and ¼
                             A Bonus

⅙ pkg vanilla-flavor ⎫
     pudding           ⎪
¼ cups whipped        ⎬ = 2¾ A Bonuses
     topping           ⎪
2 tsp brown sugar     ⎭

*220 Calories*

# Caramel-Topped Custard

*Makes 4 servings, ½ cup each.*

⅓ cup sugar
1 package (3 oz) egg custard mix
2 cups whole milk

Melt sugar in heavy skillet over medium heat, stirring constantly until golden. Pour quickly into 4 custard cups or a 2½-cup bowl; rotate quickly to coat bottoms and sides with syrup. Blend custard mix with milk in saucepan. Bring quickly to a boil, stirring constantly. (Mixture will be thin.) Pour into custard cups and chill thoroughly. Unmold.

*One serving equals about:*

| ½ cup whole milk | = | ½ Milk and ½ A Bonus |
| 4 tsp sugar | | = 1 A Bonus |
| ¼ pkg egg custard | | = 1½ A Bonuses |

*230 Calories*

# Carrot Pudding Cake

*Each loaf makes about 16 servings.*

1 package (2-layer size) yellow cake
   mix
1 package (4-serving size) vanilla-
   flavor instant pudding and pie
   filling
4 eggs
⅓ cup water
¼ cup oil
3 cups grated carrots
½ cup raisins or golden raisins,
   finely chopped
½ cup chopped walnuts or toasted
   slivered almonds
2 teaspoons cinnamon
½ teaspoon salt
   Orange Cream Cheese Frosting

Combine all ingredients except frosting in large mixer
bowl. Blend; then beat at medium speed of electric mixer
4 minutes. Pour into two greased and floured 9 × 5–inch
loaf pans. Bake at 350° for 45 to 50 minutes, or until cake
tester inserted in centers comes out clean and cakes begin
to pull away from sides of pans. *Do not underbake*. Cool
in pans about 15 minutes. Remove from pans and finish
cooling on rack. Wrap in aluminum foil and store overnight. Frost with Orange Cream Cheese Frosting.

*In high altitude areas,* use large eggs, add ¼ cup all-
purpose flour, and increase water to ¾ cup.

*Orange Cream Cheese Frosting.* Cream 1 tablespoon butter or margarine with 1 package (3 oz) cream cheese until
smooth and well blended. Gradually add 2½ cups sifted
confectioner's sugar, alternately with 1 tablespoon (about)
orange juice, beating after each addition until smooth. Stir
in 1 teaspoon grated orange rind. Makes 1¼ cups, or
enough to frost two 9-inch loaf cakes.

*Note*: One of the cakes may be wrapped and frozen for use at another time.

½-inch slice frosted cake    = 1 B Bonus

*170 Calories*


# Chocolate Cheesecake

*Makes 12 servings.*

   2 squares (2 oz) semisweet
       chocolate
   2 tablespoons water
   1 package (11 oz) unbaked
       cheesecake
   3 tablespoons sugar
   ⅓ cup butter or margarine, melted
   1½ cups cold whole milk

Melt chocolate in water in saucepan over low heat, stirring constantly until smooth. Prepare crumb mixture with sugar and butter as directed on package. Prepare filling mix with milk as directed on package; fold in chocolate. Pour into crust. Chill at least 1 hour. (Or freeze 4 hours or overnight. Let frozen cheesecake stand at room temperature at least 20 minutes before cutting.)

*One serving equals about:*

1/12 cheesecake       = 1 B Bonus

*220 Calories*

# Chocolate Mousse Pie

*Makes 12 servings.*

1½ tablespoons sugar
1 package (8 squares) semisweet
   chocolate
¼ cup water
8 eggs, separated
⅔ cup sugar
1½ teaspoons vanilla
1 teaspoon rum extract*
Dash of salt
1 cup thawed frozen whipped
   topping

Sprinkle 1½ tablespoons sugar evenly over bottom and sides of well-buttered 9-inch pie pan. Melt chocolate in water in saucepan over very low heat, stirring constantly until mixture is smooth. Remove from heat. Beat egg yolks; gradually beat in ⅔ cup sugar and continue beating until yolks are thick and light in color. Blend in melted chocolate, vanilla, and rum extract. Beat egg whites and salt until mixture will form stiff shiny peaks. Carefully fold into chocolate mixture, blending well.

Pour 4 cups of the chocolate mixture into prepared pie pan. Bake at 350° for 25 to 30 minutes or until puffed and firm. Cool 15 minutes; then chill 1 hour. (Center will fall, forming a shell.) Meanwhile, chill remaining chocolate mixture about 1½ hours. Spoon into chilled shell and chill the pie at least 3 hours. Before serving, garnish with whipped topping.

*Note*: Use clean eggs with no cracks in shells.

For ease in cutting, dip knife in hot water.

*One serving equals about:*

¹⁄₁₂ pie                          = 1 B Bonus

*220 Calories*

*Or use ¼ cup dark rum.

## Chocolate Satin Freeze

*Makes 3 cups or 6 servings.*

2 squares (2 oz) unsweetened
    chocolate
1 can (14 oz) sweetened condensed
    milk
Dash of salt
1 cup water
½ teaspoon vanilla
1 cup thawed frozen whipped
    topping

Melt chocolate in saucepan over very low heat, stirring
constantly. Blend in condensed milk and salt. Continue
to cook over very low heat 5 minutes, stirring constantly.
Remove from heat. Gradually blend in water; add vanilla.
Chill. Fold chocolate mixture into whipped topping and
pour into a 9 × 5–inch loaf pan. Freeze until frozen about
1 inch around edges. Spoon into bowl and beat until smooth
but not melted. Return to pan and freeze until firm, about
3 hours.

*One serving equals about:*

½ cup chocolate    =  ½ Milk and 1
    freeze            B Bonus

*290 Calories*

## Coffee Cream Delight

*Makes 4 servings, ½ cup each.*

1 package (4-serving size) vanilla-
    flavor pudding and pie filling
1 tablespoon instant quality coffee
1½ cups whole milk
1 cup thawed frozen whipped
    topping

Combine pudding mix, instant coffee, and milk in sauce-pan. Cook and stir over medium heat until mixture comes to a *full boil*. Pour into bowl. Place waxed paper directly on surface of hot pudding. Chill thoroughly. Then beat slowly with rotary beater until smooth. Fold in whipped topping. Spoon into dessert dishes.

*One serving equals about:*

⅓ cup whole milk  $=$  ⅓ Milk and ⅓
A Bonus

¼ pkg vanilla-flavor
   pudding and pie  $=$ 1¼ A Bonuses
   filling

¼ cup whipped
   topping  $=$ 1⅓ A Bonuses

*190 Calories*

# Easy Rice Pudding

*Makes 4 servings, ½ cup each.*

  2 cups whole milk
  ¾ cup packaged enriched precooked
     rice
  ¼ cup sugar
  1 tablespoon butter or margarine
  1 teaspoon vanilla
  ⅛ teaspoon nutmeg (optional)
  1 egg
  2 tablespoons whole milk

Bring 2 cups milk, the rice, sugar, butter, vanilla, and nutmeg to a boil in saucepan. Cook over low heat about 20 minutes, stirring frequently. Combine egg and 2 table-spoons milk; slowly add to hot rice mixture, stirring rap-idly. Pour into individual dishes. Serve warm or chilled.

*One serving equals about:*

⅓ cup cooked rice      = 1 Bread

½ cup whole milk       = ½ Milk and ½
                             A Bonus

1 tbsp sugar           = ¾ A Bonus

¾ tsp butter       ⎫
½ tbsp whole milk  ⎬ = ¾ A Bonus
¼ egg              ⎭

*240 Calories*

## Favorite Puff Pudding

*Makes about 4 cups or 8 servings.*

    ¼ cup butter or margarine
    ½ cup sugar
     1 teaspoon grated lemon rind
     2 eggs, separated
     3 tablespoons lemon juice
     2 tablespoons all-purpose flour
    ¼ cup crunchy nutlike cereal
          nuggets
     1 cup whole milk

Thoroughly cream butter with sugar and lemon rind. Add
egg yolks; beat until light and fluffy. Blend in lemon juice,
flour, cereal, and milk. (Mixture will look curdled.) Beat
egg whites until they will form stiff peaks. Fold into cereal
mixture. Pour into greased 1-quart baking dish. Set dish
in a pan of hot water. Bake at 325° for 1 hour and 15
minutes or until top springs back when lightly touched.
(Baked pudding has a cakelike layer on top with custard
below.) Serve warm or cold.

*One serving equals about:*

½ cup pudding         = 1 B Bonus

*160 Calories*

# Frozen Banana-Yogurt Dessert

*Makes 4 servings, about ⅔ cup each.*

> 1 container (8 oz) plain lowfat
>     yogurt
> 2 small bananas, mashed
> 2 tablespoons sugar
> 1 cup thawed frozen whipped
>     topping

Fold yogurt, bananas, and sugar into whipped topping, blending well. Spoon into 8- or 9-inch square pan. Freeze until firm, 4 hours or overnight. For ease in serving, transfer from freezer to refrigerator 30 minutes before serving.

*One serving equals about:*

| | |
|---|---|
| ¼ cup plain lowfat yogurt | = ¼ Milk |
| ½ small banana | = 1 Fruit |
| 1½ tsp sugar | = ½ A Bonus |
| ¼ cup whipped topping | = 1⅓ A Bonuses |

*150 Calories*

# Lemon Coconut Mousse Cake

*Makes 20 servings.*

1 package (3 oz) lemon-flavor
 pudding and pie filling
½ cup sugar
1½ cups water
3 eggs, separated
2 tablespoons butter or margarine
2 teaspoons grated lemon rind
⅓ cup sugar
1 container (4 oz) frozen whipped
 topping, thawed
9-inch commercial sponge cake
 layer
1 cup flaked coconut

Combine pudding mix, ½ cup sugar, and ¼ cup of the water in saucepan. Stir in egg yolks and remaining water. Cook and stir over medium heat until mixture comes to a *full boil*. Remove from heat; stir in butter and lemon rind. Cool to room temperature, stirring occasionally.

 Beat egg whites until foamy throughout. Gradually beat in ⅓ cup sugar; continue beating until mixture will form stiff shiny peaks. Fold in pudding; then fold in 1 cup of the whipped topping. Split cake, making 2 layers. Place 1 layer in 8- or 9-inch springform pan. Spread filling evenly over cake and top with second layer. Spread with remaining whipped topping and sprinkle with the coconut. Chill 4 hours or overnight. Remove sides of pan before serving.

*Note*: Use clean eggs with no cracks in shells.

 *One serving equals about:*

½₂₀ cake    = 1 B Bonus

*200 Calories*

# Lemon Soufflé

*Makes 4¾ cups or about 10 servings.*

1 package (3 oz) lemon-flavor
    gelatin
1 cup boiling water
¾ cup cold water
2 eggs, separated
4 tablespoons sugar
1 teaspoon grated lemon rind
1 cup thawed frozen whipped
    topping

Dissolve gelatin in boiling water. Add ½ cup of the cold water; measure ½ cup and set aside. Combine egg yolks, 2 tablespoons of the sugar, and the remaining cold water in saucepan. Cook and stir over medium heat until mixture thickens; add lemon rind. Blend into unmeasured gelatin and chill until slightly thickened. Beat egg whites until foamy throughout. Gradually beat in remaining sugar and continue beating until mixture will form stiff shiny peaks. Fold into gelatin mixture; then fold in whipped topping. Spoon into dessert dishes. Meanwhile, chill measured gelatin until slightly thickened; drizzle over creamy mixture. Chill until set, about 2 hours. Garnish with additional whipped topping, if desired.

*Note*: Use clean eggs with no cracks in shells.

*One serving equals about:*

½ cup soufflé        = 1 A Bonus

*90 Calories*

# Lemon Sours

*Makes 3 dozen.*

1 cup unsifted all-purpose flour
2 tablespoons granulated sugar
⅛ teaspoon salt
⅓ cup butter or margarine, softened
2 eggs, slightly beaten
¾ cup firmly packed dark brown
    sugar
½ cup chopped pecans or walnuts
½ cup flaked coconut
½ teaspoon vanilla
    Tart Lemon Glaze

Combine flour, granulated sugar, and salt in mixing bowl. Cut in butter until mixture resembles coarse meal. Firmly press over bottom of 8- or 9-inch square pan. Bake at 350° for 15 minutes, or until pastry is lightly browned. Meanwhile, combine eggs, brown sugar, pecans, coconut, and vanilla; mix well. Spread over pastry and bake 25 to 30 minutes longer, or until top is firm. Cool 15 minutes; then spread with Tart Lemon Glaze. Cut into bars or squares while still warm and finish cooling in pan.

*Tart Lemon Glaze.* Gradually blend 1 tablespoon lemon juice into ⅔ cup sifted confectioner's sugar in small bowl. Stir until smooth; then stir in 1 teaspoon grated lemon rind. Makes about ¼ cup glaze.

*One serving equals about:*

1 bar                    = 1 A Bonus

*70 Calories*

# Lime Chiffon Pie

*Makes 8 servings.*

1 package (4-serving size) sugar-
   free lime-flavor gelatin
1 cup boiling water
½ cup cold water
2 tablespoons lime juice
1 tablespoon grated lime rind
1 container (8 oz) frozen whipped
   topping, thawed
1 baked 8-inch pie shell, cooled

Dissolve gelatin in boiling water. Add cold water, lime juice, and rind. Chill until thickened. Blend in 3 cups whipped topping and spoon into pie shell. Chill until firm, about 3 hours. Garnish with remaining whipped topping.

*One serving equals about:*

⅛ pie                             = 1 B Bonus

*210 Calories*

# Mocha Pudding 'n Yogurt

*Makes 4 servings, about ½ cup each.*

1 cup *cold* whole milk
1 container (8 oz) coffee-flavor
   lowfat yogurt
1 package (4-serving size)
   chocolate-flavor instant
   pudding and pie filling

Combine milk and yogurt in mixing bowl. Add pudding mix and beat slowly with rotary beater until blended, about 2 minutes. Pour at once into individual dishes and let stand 5 minutes. Serve at once or chill.

*One serving equals about:*

¼ cup whole milk
¼ cup coffee-flavor          = ½ Milk and ½
    lowfat yogurt                 A Bonus

¼ pkg chocolate-
    flavor instant            = 1½ A Bonuses
    pudding

*190 Calories*

## Orange Cheesecake

*Makes 8 servings.*

¼ cup graham cracker crumbs
1 tablespoon butter or margarine
⅛ teaspoon cinnamon
3 cups (24 oz) 1% milkfat cottage
    cheese
1 package (4-serving size) sugar-
    free orange-flavor gelatin
¾ cup boiling water
2 teaspoons grated orange rind
1 teaspoon vanilla
1 container (4 oz) frozen whipped
    topping, thawed

Combine crumbs, butter, and cinnamon; set aside. Line
8-inch layer pan with waxed paper. Press cheese through
a sieve or purée in blender, a small amount at a time.
Dissolve gelatin in boiling water. Add to cheese; stir in
orange rind and vanilla. Blend in whipped topping and
pour into pan. Sprinkle evenly with crumb mixture. Chill
until firm, about 3 hours. Unmold onto serving plate and
remove paper. Garnish with orange sections if desired.

*One serving equals about:*

⅛ cheesecake            _ ⅓ Milk and 1⅓
                         =    A Bonuses

*140 Calories*

# Poached Pears

*Makes 2 servings: 1 pear and ½ tablespoon syrup each.*

2 tablespoons orange juice
1 tablespoon water
4 teaspoons firmly packed light
    brown sugar
2 teaspoons butter or margarine
½ teaspoon grated orange rind
2 medium pears, peeled

Combine orange juice, water, sugar, butter, and rind in small saucepan. Add pears. Bring liquid to a boil, basting pears frequently. Cover and poach 15 to 20 minutes or until pears are tender, turning fruit frequently. Set pears in serving dishes and bring liquid to a boil. Cook until liquid becomes syrupy, stirring frequently. Pour over pears.

*One serving equals about:*

1 medium pear        = 2 Fruit
1 tsp butter          = ½ A Bonus
2 tsp brown sugar    = ½ A Bonus

*170 Calories*

# Pot de Crème au Chocolat

*Makes about 2⅓ cups or 9 servings.*

1 package (4 oz) sweet cooking
    chocolate, broken in squares
1¼ cups half-and-half
¼ cup sugar
6 egg yolks, slightly beaten
1 teaspoon vanilla

Place chocolate, half-and-half, and sugar in saucepan. Stir constantly over low heat until chocolate is melted and mixture is smooth. Stir a small amount of the hot mixture into egg yolks, mixing well. Return to remaining hot mixture. Continue to cook and stir until slightly thickened, about 5 minutes. Add vanilla. Pour into pot de crème or demitasse cups. Chill until set.

*One serving equals about:*

¼ cup chocolate       = 1 B Bonus
    dessert

*170 Calories*

# Raspberry Sorbet

*Makes 5 cups or 10 servings.*

1 package (10 oz) frozen quick-thaw
        red raspberries in light syrup,
        thawed
1 cup cold water
1 package (3 oz) raspberry-flavor
        gelatin
1 cup sugar
2 cups boiling water

Place undrained raspberries and cold water in blender. Blend at high speed until puréed; strain to remove seeds. Dissolve gelatin and sugar in boiling water; stir in puréed raspberries. Pour into 9-inch square pan. Freeze until frozen 1 inch around edges, about 1 hour. Spoon part into blender and blend at high speed until smooth, about 30 seconds; pour into a bowl. Repeat with remaining raspberry mixture. Return all to pan and freeze until firm, about 6 hours.

*One serving equals about:*

½ cup sorbet          = 2 A Bonuses

*140 Calories*

# Southern Chocolate Pecan Pie

*Makes 16 servings.*

1 package (4 oz) sweet cooking
  chocolate
3 tablespoons butter or margarine
1 teaspoon instant quality coffee
1 cup light corn syrup
⅓ cup sugar
3 eggs, slightly beaten
1 cup coarsely chopped pecans
1 teaspoon vanilla
1 unbaked 9-inch pie shell
  Coffee-Flavored Topping
    (optional)

Melt chocolate with butter in saucepan over very low
heat, stirring constantly until smooth. Stir in coffee.
Remove from heat. Combine syrup and sugar in saucepan.
Bring to a boil over high heat, stirring until sugar is dissolved. Reduce heat and boil gently 2 minutes, stirring
occasionally. Remove from heat. Add chocolate mixture.
Pour slowly over eggs, stirring constantly. Stir in pecans
and vanilla; pour into pie shell. Bake at 375° for 45 to 50
minutes, or until filling is completely puffed across top.
Cool. Serve with Coffee-Flavored Topping.

*Coffee-Flavored Topping.* Dissolve 1 teaspoon instant
quality coffee in 1 teaspoon water. Fold into 1 cup thawed
frozen whipped topping. Makes about 1 cup.

*One serving equals about:*

¹⁄₁₆ pie with 1 tbsp     _ 1 B Bonus and
    topping               =     1 A Bonus

*260 Calories with topping*
*250 Calories without topping*

# Strawberry Bavarian

*Makes 8 servings, ½ cup each.*

1 package (3 oz) strawberry-flavor
    gelatin
1 cup boiling water
¾ cup cold water
1 container (4 oz) frozen whipped
    topping, thawed
1 cup fresh strawberries, sliced

Dissolve gelatin in boiling water. Add cold water and chill until slightly thickened. Blend in 1½ cups of the whipped topping. Chill until thickened. Fold in strawberries. Pour into 4-cup mold or individual molds. Chill until firm, about 4 hours. Unmold. Garnish with remaining whipped topping, if desired.

*One serving equals about:*

| | |
|---|---|
| ⅛ pkg strawberry gelatin | = ½ A Bonus |
| 3 tbsp whipped topping | = 1 A Bonus |
| 2 tbsp strawberries | = Negligible |

*90 Calories*

# Super Chocolate Chunk Cookies

*Makes 4 dozen.*

½ cup butter or margarine
½ cup granulated sugar
⅓ cup firmly packed light brown
     sugar
1 egg
1 teaspoon vanilla
1 cup unsifted all-purpose flour
½ teaspoon baking soda
½ teaspoon salt
1 package (8 oz) semisweet
     chocolate squares, cut into
     chunks
1 package (4 oz) sweet cooking
     chocolate, cut into chunks
¾ cup chopped walnuts

Beat butter, sugars, egg, and vanilla until light and fluffy.
Mix flour with soda and salt; blend into butter mixture.
Stir in chocolate chunks and nuts. Chill 1 hour. Drop from
teaspoon onto ungreased baking sheets, leaving 2 inches
between. Bake at 350° about 10 to 12 minutes or until
lightly browned.

*Note*: Recipe may be doubled, tripled, or quadrupled.

If dough is chilled 4 hours or overnight, let stand at room
temperature about 15 minutes before baking.

*One serving equals about:*

1 cookie                    = 1 A Bonus

*90 Calories*

# Trifle Treat

*Makes 7 cups or 14 servings.*

1 package (4-serving size) vanilla-
     or French-vanilla–flavor
     instant pudding and pie filling
2 cups *cold* whole milk
1 container (4 oz) frozen whipped
     topping, thawed
4 cups pound cake cubes
½ cup orange juice
¼ cup sherry wine
2 tablespoons water
⅓ cup raspberry or strawberry
     preserves
½ cup soft macaroon crumbs

Prepare pudding mix with milk as directed on package for
pudding; fold in 1 cup of the whipped topping and set
aside. Place cake cubes in a 1½-quart serving bowl. Combine orange juice and wine; sprinkle over cake. Stir water
into preserves and spoon over cake. Sprinkle with macaroon crumbs. Add pudding mixture, covering cake cubes
completely. Chill at least 2 hours. Garnish with remaining
whipped topping.

*One serving equals about:*

½ cup dessert          = 1 B Bonus

*180 Calories*

# Vanilla Pudding 'n Yogurt

*Makes 4 servings, about ½ cup each.*

1 cup *cold* whole milk
1 container (8 oz) lowfat plain
    yogurt
1 package (4-serving size) vanilla-
    flavor instant pudding and pie
    filling

Combine milk and yogurt in mixing bowl. Add pudding
mix and beat slowly with rotary beater until blended,
about 2 minutes. Pour at once into individual dishes and
let stand 5 minutes. Serve at once or chill.

*One serving equals about:*

| | |
|---|---|
| ¼ cup whole milk ⎫ | = ½ Milk and ⅓ |
| ¼ cup lowfat plain ⎬ | A Bonus |
| yogurt ⎭ | |
| ¼ pkg vanilla-flavor | = 1½ A Bonuses |
| instant pudding | |

*170 Calories*

# Zabaglione

*Makes about 3 cups or 6 servings.*

1 package (4-serving size) vanilla-
    flavor pudding and pie filling
1½ cups whole milk
¼ cup sherry wine
2 egg whites
    Dash of salt

Combine pudding mix and milk in saucepan. Cook and
stir over medium heat until mixture comes to a *full boil*.
Remove from heat and stir in wine. Beat egg whites and

salt until they will form stiff peaks. Gradually fold in hot pudding. Pour into individual dessert dishes. Serve warm.

*Note*: Use clean eggs with no cracks in shells.

> *One serving equals about:*
>
> ½ cup pudding          $=$   ¼ Milk and 1
>                                        A Bonus
>
> *100 Calories*

# Dessert Sauces/Toppings

## Crisp Dessert Topping

*Makes about 2½ cups or 13 servings.*

2 tablespoons butter or margarine
1 cup 40% bran flakes or crisp
    whole wheat flakes
⅔ cup flaked coconut
¼ cup chopped nuts
¼ cup firmly packed brown sugar
½ teaspoon cinnamon

Melt butter in skillet; add remaining ingredients. Cook and stir over medium heat until mixture is golden brown. Cool. Sprinkle on ice cream, pudding, fruit, yogurt, cottage cheese, or frosted cake. Leftover topping can be stored in tightly covered container up to 2 weeks.

*One serving equals about:*

3 tbsp topping      = 1 A Bonus

*75 Calories*

## Regal Chocolate Sauce

*Makes about 1 cup or 16 servings.*

   2 squares (2 oz) unsweetened
        chocolate
   6 tablespoons water
   ½ cup sugar
        Dash of salt
   3 tablespoons butter or margarine
   ¼ teaspoon vanilla

Heat chocolate and water in saucepan over very low heat, stirring constantly until chocolate is melted and smooth. Add sugar and salt. Continue to cook and stir about 5 minutes, or until sugar is dissolved and mixture is very slightly thickened. Remove from heat. Add butter and vanilla; stir until sauce is smooth.

*One serving equals about:*
1 tbsp sauce                = 1 A Bonus

*60 Calories*

## Silken Raspberry Sauce

*Makes about 1¾ cups sauce or 14 servings.*

   1 package (10 oz) frozen quick-thaw
        red raspberries in light syrup
   ½ cup currant jelly
   2 tablespoons orange liqueur

Hold quick-thaw pouch under hot tap water until fruit is loosened from pouch but not thawed. Empty fruit into blender. Add jelly and liqueur. Cover and blend at high speed until smooth. Serve over ice cream, sherbet, or fruit.

*One serving equals about:*
2 tbsp sauce                = 1 A Bonus

*50 Calories*

## Beverages

### Mulled Cranberry Punch

*Makes 18 servings, ½ cup each.*

1 envelope tropical punch–flavor
    sugar-free soft drink mix
5 whole cloves
1 stick cinnamon
6 cups boiling water
3 cups cranberry juice cocktail

Combine soft drink mix and spices in heatproof plastic or glass punch bowl or pitcher. Add boiling water and stir until soft drink mix is dissolved. Add cranberry juice cocktail; let stand about 10 minutes. Remove spices and serve punch warm.

*One serving equals about:*

⅓ cup sugar-free
    soft drink      = Negligible

⅙ cup cranberry
    juice cocktail    = ½ Fruit

*25 Calories*

# South Seas Cooler

*Makes about 4²/₃ cups or 12 servings, about ¹/₃ cup each.*

    1 tub lemonade-flavor sugar-free
            drink mix
    1¼ cups water
    2 cups unsweetened pineapple juice
    ²/₃ cup cream of coconut
    ¾ cup vodka or rum
    Crushed ice

Dissolve drink mix in water in large plastic or glass pitcher.
Add pineapple juice, cream of coconut, and vodka. Chill.
Serve over crushed ice.

*One serving equals about:*

| | |
|---|---|
| ⅙ cup pineapple juice | = ½ Fruit |
| 2½ tsp cream of coconut | = ½ A Bonus |
| ½ oz vodka | = ½ A Bonus |

*110 Calories with vodka*
*70 Calories without vodka*

# Miscellaneous

## Breakfast Bars

*Makes 8 servings.*

6 cups crisp whole wheat flakes
4 eggs
⅓ cup chopped pecans (16 halves)
¼ cup firmly packed brown sugar
¼ cup butter or margarine, melted
1 cup part-skim ricotta cheese
½ cup chopped dates
1 tablespoon granulated sugar

Combine cereal, 3 eggs, the nuts, brown sugar, and butter in large bowl; toss to blend. Measure 2 cups and set aside. Press remaining mixture over bottom of greased 9-inch square pan. Combine cheese, remaining egg, dates, and granulated sugar. Spread evenly over mixture in pan; then sprinkle with reserved cereal mixture. Bake at 350° for 30 minutes. Cool; then cut into 8 bars.

*One serving equals about:*

| | |
|---|---|
| ¾ cup whole wheat flakes | = 1½ Bread |
| ½ egg | = ¼ Meat |
| 2 pecan halves | = ½ A Bonus |
| 2 tsp sugars | = ½ A Bonus |
| 1½ tsp butter | = 1 A Bonus |
| 2 tbsp part-skim ricotta cheese | = ½ Milk |
| 1 tbsp dates | = ¼ Fruit |

*320 Calories*

# Cottage Cheese—Dill Dip

*Makes 10 servings, ¼ cup each.*

1 container (16 oz) 1% milkfat
    medium- or small-curd cottage
    cheese
1 container (8 oz) plain yogurt
¼ cup finely chopped onion*
1 tablespoon chopped fresh
    dillweed*
⅛ teaspoon white or black pepper

Place all ingredients in small bowl. Stir to combine thoroughly. Chill at least 1 hour. Serve as dip for fresh vegetable pieces, such as cauliflower and broccoli florets, cherry tomatoes, carrot sticks, and cucumber slices.

*One serving equals about:*

$$\frac{\text{¼ cup 1\% milkfat}}{\text{cottage cheese}} = \frac{\text{¼ Milk and ¼}}{\text{A Bonus}}$$

1½ tbsp plain yogurt = Negligible

*50 Calories*

*Or substitute ½ teaspoon garlic powder OR 3 tablespoons prepared horseradish for the onion and dillweed.

# References

1. Adam, J., T. W. Bestrand, and O. G. Edholm. Weight changes in young men. *J. Physiol.* (Lond.), *156*: 38, 1961.

2. Ahrens, R. A., C. L. Bishop, and C. D. Berdanier. Effect of age and dietary carbohydrate source on the response of rats and forced exercise. *J. Nutr.* *102*: 241, 1972.

3. Andik, I., J. Bank, I. Moring, and G. Y. Szegvari. The effect of exercise on the intake and selection of food in the rat. *Act. Physiol. Hung.* *5*: 457, 1954.

4. Apfelbaum, M., J. Bostsarron, and D. Lacatis. Effect of caloric restriction and excessive caloric intake on energy expenditure. *Am. J. Clin. Nutr.* *24*: 1405, 1971.

5. Bennett, W. and J. Gurin. *The Dieter's Dilemma*. Basic Books, New York, 1982.

6. Bernstein, R., J. Thornton, A. Redmond, F. X. Pi-Sunyer, J. Wang, M. Yang, and T. Van Itallie. Physiologic changes after a conservative weight loss program. *IV Int. Congr. Obesity.* New York, October, 1983.

7. Boileau, R. A., E. R. Buskirk, D. H. Horstman, J. Mendey, and W. C. Nichols. Body composition changes in obese and lean men during physical conditioning. *Med. Sci. Sports 3*: 183, 1971.

8. Bradfield, R. B., D. E. Curtis, and S. Margen. Effect of activity on caloric response of obese women. *Am. J. Clin. Nutr.* *21*: 1208, 1968.

9. Bray, G. A. Effect of caloric restriction on energy expenditure in obese patients. *Lancet ii*: 397, 1969.

10. Bray, G. A. The energetics of obesity. *Med. and Sci. in Sports and Exercise.* 15 no. 1, 1983: 32–40.

11. Bray, G. A., B. J. Whipp, and S. N. Koyal. The acute effects of food intake on energy expenditure during cycle ergometry. *Am. J. Clin. Nutr.* *27*: 254, 1974.

12. Brooks, McC. and E. F. Lambert. A study of the effect of limitation of food intake and the method of feeding on the rate of weight gain during hypothalamic obesity in the albino rat. *Am. J. Physiol.* *147*: 717, 1946.

13. Brownell, K. D. The psychology and physiology of obesity: implications for screening and treatment. *J. of the Am. Dietetic Assoc. 84*. No. 4, Apr. 1984: 406–413.

14. Buskirk, E. R., R. H. Thompson, L. Lutwak, and G. D. Whedon. Energy balance of obese patients during weight reduction: influence of diet restriction and exercise. *Ann. NY Acad. Sci. 110*: 918, 1963.

15. Cohn, C. and D. Joseph. Influence of body weight and body fat on appetite of "normal" lean and obese rats. *Yale J. Biol. Med. 34*: 589, 1962.

16. Collier, G., A. I. Leshner, and R. L. Squibb. Dietary self-selection in active and non-active rats. *Physiol. Behav. 4*: 79, 1969.

17. Crews, E. L., K. W. Fuge, L. B. Oscai, J. O. Holloszy, and R. E. Shank. Weight, food intake, and body composition effects of exercise and of protein deficiency. *Am. J. Physiol. 216*: 359, 1969.

18. Davis, J. R., A. R. Tagliaferro, R. Kentzer, J. Gerardo, J. Nichols, and J. Wheeler. Variations in dietary-induced thermogenesis and body fatness with aerobic capacity. *Eur. J. Appl. Physiol. Occup. Physiol. 50*: 319, 1983.

19. Davis, J. R., R. Kertzer, and A. R. Tagliaferro. Dietary-induced thermogenesis enhanced by endurance training. *Fed. Proc. 41*: 715, #2604, 1982.

20. DeVries, H. A. and D. E. Gray. Aftereffects of exercise upon resting metabolism rate. *Res. Quarterly 34*: 314, 1963.

21. Donahue, C. P., Jr., D. H. Lin, D. S. Kirschenbaum and R. E. Keesey. Metabolic Consequences of Dieting and Exercise in the Treatment of Obesity. *J. of Consulting and Clinical Psychology*: Vol. 52, No. 5, 827–836, 1984.

22. Edholm, O. G., J. G. Fletcher, E. M. Widdowson, and R. A. McCance. The energy expenditure and food intake of individual men. *Brit. J. Nutr. 9*: 286, 1955.

23. Epstein, L. H., B. J. Masek, and W. R. Marshall. A nutritionally based school program for control of eating in obese children. *Behav. Ther. 9*: 766, 1978.

24. Forbes, G. B. and J. C. Reina. Adult lean body mass declines with age: some longitudinal observations. *Metabolism 19*: 653, 1970.

25. Garrow, J. S. *Energy Balance and Obesity in Man.* 2 ed. Elsevier, Amsterdam, 1978.

26. Gleeson, M., J. F. Brown, J. J. Waring, and M. J. Stock. The effects of physical exercise on metabolic rate and dietary induced thermogenesis. *Brit. J. Nutr. 47*: 173, 1982.

27. Grande, F., J. T. Anderson, and A. Keys. Changes of basal metabolic rate in man in semistarvation and refeeding. *Am. J. Physiol.* *12*: 230, 1958.

28. Gwinup. G. Effect of exercise alone on the weight of obese women. *Arch. Intern. Med. 135*: 676, 1975.

29. Harris, R. B. S. and R. J. Martin. Lipostatic theory of energy balance: concepts and signals. *Nutr. and Behavior. 1*: 253–275, 1984.

30. Harris, R. B. S. and R. J. Martin. Recovery of body weight from below "set point" in mature female rats. *J. Nutr. 114*: 1143–1150, 1984.

31. Hill, J., J. Davis, and T. Tagliaferro. Effects of a supermarket diet and exercise training on food intake, body weight, body fat, and dietary-induced thermogenesis in adult female rats. *Fed. Proc. 41*: 401, #765, 1982.

32. Hill, J. O., J. R. Davis, and A. R. Tagliaferro. Effects of diet and exercise training on thermogenesis in adult female rats. *Physiol. Behav. 31*: 133, 1983.

33. Hill, J. O., S. B. Heymsfield, C. McManus III, and M. DiGirolamo. Meal size and thermic response to feed in male subjects as a function of maximum aerobic capacity. *Metab. 33*: 743, 1984.

34. Ingle, D. J. A simple means of producing obesity in the rat. *Endocrinology 72*: 604, 1949.

35. Johnson, D. and E. J. Brenick. Therapeutic fasting in morbid obesity: long-term follow-up. *Arch. Intern. Med. 137*: 1381, 1977.

36. Katahn, M. *Beyond Diet: The 28-Day Metabolic Breakthrough Plan.* W. W. Norton & Company, New York, 1984.

37. Katch, V. L., R. Martin, and J. Martin. Effects of exercise intensity on food consumption in the male rat. *Am J. Clin. Nutr. 32*: 1401, 1979.

38. Keesey, R. E. A set point analysis of the regulation of body weight. In A. J. Stunkard, ed. *Obesity.* W. B. Saunders, New York, 1980.

39. Keesey, R. E. Metabolic defense of the body weight set point. In A. J. Stunkard and E. Stellan, *Eating and Its Disorders*, p. 87, Raven Press, New York, 1984.

40. Kenrick, M. M., M. F. Ball, and J. J. Canary. Exercise and weight reduction in obesity. *Arch. Phys. Med. Rehabil. 53*: 323, 1972.

41. Keys, A., H. L. Taylor, and F. Grande. Basal metabolism and age of adult man. *Metabolism 22*: 579, 1973.

42. Keys, A., J. Brozek, A. Henschel, O. Mickelsen, and H. L. Taylor. *The Biology of Human Starvation*. 2 vols. University of Minnesota Press, Minneapolis, 1950.

43. Khosha, T., and W. Z. Billewicz. Measurement of changes in body weight. *Brit. J. Nutr. 18*: 227, 1964.

44. Leibel, R. L., and J. Hirsch. Diminished energy requirements in reduced-obese patients. *Metab. 33*. no. 2, Feb. 1984.

45. Leon, A. S., J. Conrad, D. B. Hunninghake, and R. Serfass. Effects of a vigorous walking program on body composition, and carbohydrate and lipid metabolism of obese young men. *Am. J. Clin. Nutr. 32*: 1776, 1979.

46. Mayer, J., N. B. Marshall, J. J. Vitale, J. H. Christensen, M. B. Mashayekhi, and F. J. Stare. Exercise, food intake, and body weight in normal rats and genetically obese adult mice. *Am. J. Physiol. 177*: 544, 1954.

47. Mayer, J., P. Roy and K. P. Mitra. Relation between caloric intake, body weight, and physical work: studies in an industrial male population in West Bengal. *Am. J. Clin. Nutr. 4*: 169, 1956.

48. McCance, R. A. Food, growth and time. *Lancet ii*: 671, 1962.

49. Miller, D. S., P. Mumford, and M. J. Stock. Gluttony 2. Thermogenesis in overeating man. *Am. J. Clin. Nutr. 20*: 1223, 1967.

50. Moody, D. L., J. Kollias, and E. R. Buskirk. The effect of a moderate exercise program on body weight and skinfold thickness in overweight college women. *Med. Sci. Sports 1*: 75, 1969.

51. Moody, D. L., J. H. Wilmore, R. N. Girandola, and J. P. Royce. The effects of a jogging program on the body composition of normal and obese high school girls. *Med. Sci. Sports 4*: 210, 1972.

52. Nance, D. W., B. Bromley, R. J. Barnard, and R. Gorski. Sexually dimorphic effects of forced exercise on food intake and body weight in the rat. *Physiol. Behav. 9*: 155, 1977.

53. Nikoletseas, M. M. Exercise-induced sucrose suppression in the rat. *Physiol. Behav. 26*: 145, 1981.

54. Nisbitt, R. E. Hunger, obesity, and the ventromedial hypothalamus. *Psychol. Rev. 79*.: 433, 1972.

55. Oscai, L. B. and J. O. Holloszy. Effects of weight changes produced by exercise, food restriction, or overeating on body composition. *J. Clin. Invest. 48*: 2124, 1969.

56. Passmore, R. and R. E. Johnson. Some metabolic changes following prolonged moderate exercise. *Metabolism 9*: 452, 1960.

57. Pitts, G. C., L. S. Bull, and J. A. Wakefield. Exercise with force feeding in the rat. *Am. J. Physiol. 227*: 341, 1974.

58. Robinson, M. D., and P. E. Watson. Day to day variations in body weight of young women. *Brit. J. Nutr. 19*: 225, 1965.

59. Rolls, B. J. and E. A. Rowe. Exercise and the development and persistence of dietary obesity in male and female rats. *Physiol. Behav. 23*: 241, 1979.

60. Schultz, C. K., E. Bernauer, P. A. Mole, H. R. Superko, and J. S. Stern. Effects of severe caloric restriction and moderate exercise on basal metabolic rate and hormonal status in adult humans. *Fed. Proc. 39*: 3, 1980.

61. Sims, E. A. H., E. Danforth, E. S. Horton, G. A. Bray, J. A. Glennan, and L. B. Salans. Endocrine and metabolic effects of experimental obesity in man. *Recent Progress in Hormone Research 29*: 457, 1973.

62. Sims, E. A. H. et al. Experimental obesity in man. *Transactions of the Association of American Physicians 81*: 153, 1968.

63. Spiegel, T. A. Caloric regulation of food intake in man. *J. Comp. Physiol. Psychol. 84*: 24, 1973.

64. Stunkard, A. J. Anorectic agents lower a body weight set point. *Life Sci. 30*: 2043, 1982.

65. Stunkard, A. J. Behavioral treatments of obesity: failure to maintain weight loss. In R. B. Stuart, ed. *Behavioral Self-Management.* Brunner, New York, 1977.

66. Stunkard A. J. Physical activity and obesity. *Susmen LIIK-UNTALAAKETIEDE 2*: 99–111, 1983. (*Finnish Sports and Exercise Medicine*).

67. Thompson, J. K., G. J. Jarvie, B. B. Lahey, and K. J. Cureton. Exercise and obesity: etiology, physiology, and intervention. *Psychol. Bull. 91*: 55, 1982.

68. Warwick, P. M. and J. S. Garrow. The effect of addition of exercise to a regime of dietary restriction on weight loss, nitrogen balance, resting metabolic rate and spontaneous physical activity in three obese women in a metabolic ward. *Int. J. Obesity 5*: 25, 1981.

69. Woo, R., J. S. Garrow, and F. X. Pi-Sunyer. Effect of exercise on spontaneous caloric intake in obesity. *Am. J. Clin. Nutr. 36*: 470, 1982a.

70. Woo, R., J. S. Garrow, and F. X. Pi-Sunyer. Voluntary food intake during prolonged exercise in obese women. *Am. J. Clin. Nutr. 36*: 478, 1982b.

# ₩₦ INDEX

# ₩¶¶ RECIPES

# About the Author

Dr. Gilbert A. Leveille was born in Massachusetts in 1934. He received a bachelor's degree from the University of Massachusetts and both an M.S. and a Ph.D. in nutrition and biochemistry from Rutgers University.

Dr. Leveille is director of nutrition and health sciences at the General Foods Corporation. He was appointed to the position in 1980 after serving for nearly ten years as chairman of the department of food science and human nutrition at Michigan State University.

He is past president of the Institute of Food Technologists. He has served as president of the National Nutrition Consortium and chairman of the Food and Nutrition Board of the National Research Council of the National Academy of Sciences. He lectures widely and has published more than three hundred scientific papers.

At General Foods, Dr. Leveille is responsible for research in nutrition, physiology, dental health, and toxicology. He led a research team in the three-year development of the Setpoint Diet. He contributes to corporate policy regarding nutrition and health and participates in the verification of health-related claims in product labeling and advertising.

# Ballantine Books:
# A Dieter's Best Friend